This edition published in Australia in 2009 by
New Holland Publishers (Australia) Pty Ltd
Sydney • Auckland • London • Cape Town

1/66 Gibbes Street, Chatswood NSW 2067 Australia
www.newholland.com.au
218 Lake Road Northcote Auckland 0746 New Zealand
86 Edgware Road London W2 2EA United Kingdom
80 McKenzie Street Cape Town 8001 South Africa

First edition published 1990

National Library of Australia Cataloguing-in-Publication details:

    Roberts, Christine.
    Diabetes : eat and enjoy / Christine
          Roberts, Margaret Cox and Jennifer Mcdonald.
    4th ed.
    9781741108149 (pbk.)
    Diabetes--Diet therapy--Recipes.
    Other Authors/Contributors:
          McDonald, Jennifer
          Cox, Margaret.
    616.4620654

Publisher: Fiona Schultz
Publishing Manager: Lliane Clarke
Project Editor: Diane Jardine
Designer: Hayley Norman
Additional food photography: Graeme Gillies
Production Manager: Olga Dementiev
Printer: Everbest Printing Co Ltd, China

10 9 8 7 6 5 4 3 2 1

DIABETES:
Eat & Enjoy
FOURTH EDITION

Christine Roberts   Margaret Cox   Jennifer McDonald

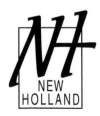

NEW
HOLLAND

Contents

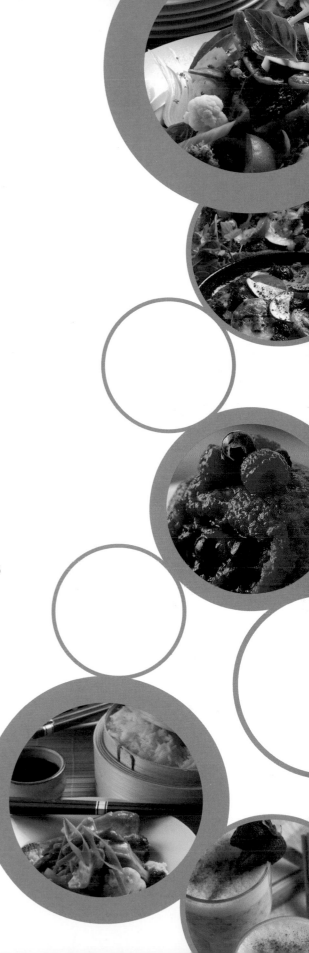

4   Introduction
7   **About diabetes**
10 Types of diabetes
14 Recognising diabetes
15 **Management of diabetes**
18 Food for health and diabetes
36 Medication for diabetes
37 Illness and diabetes
39 Hypoglycaemia
42 Diabetes and coeliac disease
45 Pregnancy and diabetes
46 Childhood and adolescence
48 Diabetes and older people
50 Vegetarians with diabetes
53 Exercise, sport and diabetes
56 **Eating to suit your needs**
56 Eating out
59 Occasional treats
60 Travelling across time zones
61 Shift work
62 **Making sense of food labels**
62 The ingredients list
63 The nutrition panel
64 Packaging claims
67 Artificial and alternative sweetners
68 **Recipes**
72 Breakfasts
78 Snacks
88 Lunches and light meals
120 Main meals
225 Desserts and sweet treats
248 Nibbles and party foods
260 Special occasion meals
274 **Food value lists**
284 Recipe Index
286 Index

Introduction

Over the years we have provided information about diet, cooking and eating, to many hundreds of people with diabetes. We have been aware of a need for easy to read, straightforward and up-to-date information on food and diabetes, the effects food has on diabetes management, and on ways to plan and prepare interesting and delicious meals.

This book explains in simple terms the relationship between diabetes and food, provides guidelines for good management and includes delicious and healthy recipes that are ideal not only for those with diabetes, but for the whole family. Through this book we hope that you will develop more confidence in your ability to maintain good health and to eat with enjoyment.

The information in this book is current at the time of publication. Research into diabetes continues and areas of management may undergo further change.

Acknowledgements

There are a number of people who have helped and encouraged us in the writing of this book.

We would like, firstly, to acknowledge Diabetes Australia State and Territory organisations for their support.

We'd especially like to thank Naomi Roberts BSc, MND, Dietitian for her invaluable advice and editorial input, Rebecca Hall, student dietitian for her invaluable assistance with the analysis of the recipes and Narelle Harvey, Registered Nurse, Credentialled Diabetes Educator, for her expert assistance with updating the clinical information in this new edition.

We thank also our editors and publishers including Diane Jardine and Fiona Schultz of New Holland Publishers who have helped make this fourth edition of *Diabetes: Eat & Enjoy* possible.

Most importantly, we thank our families, and especially our husbands—Noel Roberts, Jack Cox and Michael Hall. Without their support, patience, encouragement and understanding, we could never have completed *Diabetes Eat & Enjoy*.

Christine Roberts, Margaret Cox, Jennifer McDonald

About the authors

Christine Roberts is an Australian Dietitian who is also registered in the UK. Most recently she has worked at the University of Surrey, United Kingdom as Dietetic Programme Development Consultant and in teaching dietetics and nutrition. As an Accredited Practising Dietitian, she worked for many years as Head Dietitian at St Georges Hospital and amalgamated health services in Melbourne, as the Director of Melbourne Dietetic Centre and as a Consultant Dietitian to hospitals, commercial organisations and in private practice. Over this time she has had much involvement with the management of diabetes and has co-authored a number of papers and other publications on diet and diabetes.

Margaret Cox has worked for many years as a Dietitian in community health in Victoria. Her special interest in all aspects of diabetes and its management began with a period as Senior Dietitian at the International Diabetes Institute in Melbourne, and has continued throughout her career. Development of diabetes group education programs, working with individuals and families, and establishing close working relationships with Diabetes educators to educate, support, and assist people with diabetes, and to educate the public about diabetes, have remained a major focus of her work. Margaret has co-authored several papers and other publications on diet and diabetes. She currently works as a Dietitian with the North Eastern Victorian Division of General Practice.

Jennifer McDonald is an Accredited Practising Dietitian (A.P.D.) and is currently the coordinator of the Percutaneous Endoscopic Gastrostomy (PEG) Outreach Service at Southern Health. She is a Consultant Dietitian to various international pharmaceutical companies. As well as these roles she works in private practice with Diabetes Specialists at the Box Hill Diabetes and Endocrine Service and at the Jean Hailes Foundation for Women's Health. Over the years, together with other top researchers specialising in diabetes, she has co-authored a number of scientific papers dealing with diet and diabetes. She has also been involved in writing many publications for people with diabetes.

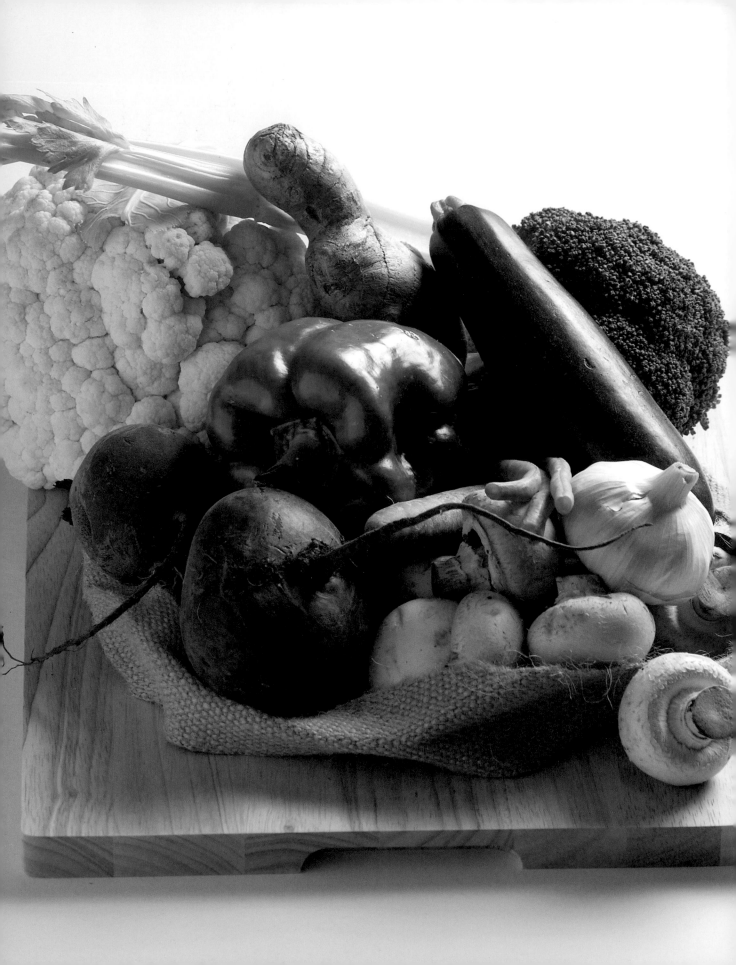

About
diabetes

Diabetes mellitus is not new. It may be as old as humanity and has been with us throughout recorded history. It was not until 1921 when insulin was discovered that the lives of people with diabetes were saved and only in very recent years have we understood diabetes better and had access to more effective management.

Diabetes is one of the fastest growing disease epidemics in human history and can lead to increased health problems and premature death if not effectively managed.

The number of people with diabetes in Australia has doubled between 1989 and 2005. The figures are disturbing:

- 275 Australians develop diabetes every day
- approximately 100,000 adult Australians are diagnosed each year
- currently more than 800,000 Australians have been diagnosed with diabetes
- it is estimated that for every person diagnosed there is another not diagnosed
- by 2020, it is predicted that at least two million Australians will be diagnosed with diabetes
- in addition, many more Australians have a condition known as pre-diabetes
- nearly 1 in 4 adult Australians over 25 years have diabetes or pre-diabetes
- it is estimated that currently 3.2 million Australians have either diabetes or pre-diabetes.

Diabetes means too much sugar in the blood

'Diabetes' comes from the ancient Greek word for 'siphon', referring to the large amount of sugar-containing urine passed by people with poorly managed diabetes, and 'mellitus' for the characteristic sweet taste of the urine.

Diabetes (more accurately 'diabetes mellitus') is simply too much sugar in the blood. This sugar is in the form of glucose. Diabetes occurs when the system which controls the amount of glucose in the blood no longer works properly.

Glucose comes from the food we eat

Glucose comes from the sugars and starches in the foods we eat. When we eat sugars and starches, our bodies convert it into glucose.

Foods rich in carbohydrate sugars and starches include:

- breads, cereals and biscuits
- pulses (such as dried peas, beans and lentils)
- starchy vegetables (such as potatoes)
- rice and pasta
- fruit
- milk
- sugar
- foods with sugar added, such as cakes, sweet biscuits, confectionery, soft drinks and canned fruit.

The digestive system breaks down carbohydrate sugars and starches to make **glucose** and other sugars. The sugars are then absorbed into the bloodstream directly from the digestive tract (gut).

The body uses glucose for fuel

The blood carries the glucose to the cells of your body tissues (for instance, your lungs, heart, kidneys and muscles) where it is used as fuel (energy). The only way the glucose can get into the cells is with the help of a hormone called **insulin**.

Insulin helps lower the blood glucose level

Insulin is produced by the pancreas. After you have eaten, digested and absorbed food containing carbohydrate, the amount of glucose in your blood increases. In response to this, the pancreas releases insulin into your blood to carry the glucose into the cells. This lowers the glucose level in the blood so it returns to where it was before the meal.

If you don't have diabetes, your blood glucose level never goes too high or too low, no matter how much or how little carbohydrate you eat. The system balances itself.

High blood glucose levels cause symptoms of diabetes

When the body produces little or no insulin, or the insulin it does produce is unable to carry glucose into your body cells, you develop diabetes.

With your normal glucose regulating system out of order, the level of glucose in the blood keeps increasing. When it reaches a certain level, the body flushes the extra glucose out of your body via your urine.

A high blood glucose may cause all or some of the following symptoms:

- the passing of large amounts of urine (polyuria) particularly at night time (nocturia) as a way of getting rid of the excess sugar

- thirst, a dry mouth and excessive drinking (polydypsia) in response to the large urine output
- excessive tiredness due to the lack of available fuel to the cells
- weight loss—because the normal fuel (glucose) is not available and the body uses fat stores
- infections, slow wound healing and itchiness resulting from bacteria feeding on the extra glucose in blood and urine
- blurring of vision as the high blood glucose level alters the ability of the eye to focus.

A high blood glucose level is known as hyperglycaemia, from 'hyper', meaning excessive and 'glycaemia' for sugar in the blood.

Where to go for more information about diabetes

Following are some recommended sources of information about diabetes.

Accredited Practising Dietitians (APD)

APDs are the experts in all aspects of dietary advice to suit your lifestyle. Many are also Credentialled Diabetes Educators (CDEs).

- Visit the Dietitians' Association of Australia website at www.daa.asn.au
- Look under 'Dietitian' in the Yellow Pages or other telephone directory
- Ask your local doctor if he or she can refer you to a dietitian
- Contact your community health centre
- Telephone your local hospital
- Enquire at your state or Commonwealth health department

Diabetes Australia

Diabetes Australia is the nation's leading diabetes consumer organisation providing a unique partnership between consumers—the people with diabetes—diabetes research organisations, doctors and other health professionals with a special interest in diabetes.

Visit Diabetes Australia's website www.diabetesaustralia.com.au which has links to each State and Territory website. Look for Diabetes Australia in your telephone directory.

Diabetes Australia State and Territory organisations provide dietary services, educational literature, free magazines, product discounts for members and other benefits, services for children with diabetes, support groups and access to the National Diabetes Services Scheme (NDSS) an Australian Government initiative providing free syringes, pen needles and insulin pump consumables plus subsidised blood glucose strips and urine testing strips.

The Australian Diabetes Educator's Association (ADEA)

The ADEA is a leading organisation for health professionals providing diabetes education and care. Visit the ADEA website www.adea.com.au to find your closest CDE. A CDE can assist you in understanding diabetes and navigating lifestyle change. They can help you establish networks with others with diabetes and advise on monitoring blood glucose and using the results of this to improve diabetes management.

Other websites and places to seek information

- www.healthyactive.gov.au for healthy eating, physical activity and overweight issues
- for healthy eating www.health.gov.au
- The Heart Foundation www.heartfoundation.org.au has information on general healthy eating, weight management, reducing risk of heart disease and recipes.

Types of diabetes

There are three main types of diabetes mellitus:

- Type 1 diabetes
- Type 2 diabetes
- Gestational diabetes

There are two conditions linked to the development of Type 2 diabetes:

- Impaired fasting glucose (IFG)
- Impaired glucose tolerance (IGT)

Other types of diabetes mellitus may result from genetic abnormalities, or certain triggers such as injury to the pancreas, or certain medications used to treat other conditions. There is also another type of diabetes known as diabetes insipidus where symptoms of increased urinary output and thirst occur. This is unrelated to diabetes mellitus.

Type 1 diabetes

Type 1 diabetes used to be called Insulin-Dependent Diabetes Mellitus—IDDM or Juvenile onset diabetes. This type of diabetes results from damage or deterioration of the pancreas leading to a complete lack of insulin production. Approximately 10–15% of Australians with diabetes have this type of diabetes. It can occur at any age but usually develops in people under 30 years of age.

Risk factors

The risk factors and cause for Type 1 diabetes are unknown. Type 1 diabetes can occur at any age but usually develops in people under 30 years of age. Although the cause is still unknown, a strong family history of Type 1 diabetes and environmental factors, such as a viral infection, appear to lead to the destruction of the insulin producing cells of the pancreas. Symptoms usually appear quickly and severely. If not treated promptly, your blood glucose level rises excessively. As the glucose cannot get into the cells, your body quickly begins to burn up its fat stores. The breath develops a sweet sickly smell and vomiting, dehydration and drowsiness may occur. Left untreated, you will eventually pass into a coma.

Treatment

Treatment for Type 1 diabetes is a combination of:
- insulin
- the healthy eating pattern we present in this book.

Type 2 diabetes

Type 2 diabetes used to be called Non-Insulin-Dependent Diabetes Mellitus—NIDDM or Mature onset diabetes. This is the major type of diabetes. It affects 7.5% of all Australians over 25 years of age and accounts for about 85–90% of all cases of diabetes in Australia. It occurs when the pancreas cannot make enough insulin ('insulin insufficiency') or the body is unable to use it properly ('insulin resistance').

Type 2 diabetes usually develops slowly. Symptoms, if any, are likely to be less extreme than with Type 1 diabetes. The only sign may be a high blood glucose level (hyperglycaemia) which is picked up on routine medical review, eye examination by Ophthalmologist or eye specialist, or through screening for pre-diabetes or diabetes.

Risk factors

Type 2 diabetes usually develops in people over the age of forty. However, as the population becomes less active and more obese, it is becoming more common in younger people including children less than 12 years old. A number of factors may increase the likelihood of developing Type 2 diabetes.

Some of these cannot be changed but others may relate to lifestyle and, although not always easy to do, can be changed. Risk factors that cannot be changed include:
- family history
- age, with risk increasing as we get older

- ethnic predisposition in indigenous Australians (mainland and Torres Straits Islands) and people from the Indian subcontinent and Chinese or Pacific Islander background
- presence of impaired fasting glucose or impaired glucose tolerance
- women with a history of gestational diabetes or where they have given birth to an infant over 4.5 kilograms (9 pounds).
- women with polycystic ovarian syndrome
- people with clinical cardiovascular disease.

Risk factors that can be changed include:
- being overweight, particularly where excess weight is carried around the waistline
- high blood pressure
- raised blood fat levels
- inactivity
- unhealthy eating habits
- stress or depression
- alcohol abuse.

Treatment

Treatment for Type 2 diabetes involves a healthy eating plan and exercise. For the overweight person with this type of diabetes, losing weight is the most important part of treatment. If this is not enough to manage the blood glucose then oral medication or insulin may be given.

Even with well-managed diabetes, insulin or extra oral medication may be needed during periods of illness, emotional distress or after surgery. Type 2 diabetes is a progressive condition and with time, the pancreatic function of people with diabetes will deteriorate. Despite a healthy lifestyle, insulin (often in combination with oral medication) will be needed to manage the blood glucose. Although the deterioration in some cases may be slow, around 50% of people will require insulin within 10 years of diagnosis.

Gestational diabetes

Diabetes in pregnancy occurs in around 5.5–8% of all pregnancies and usually develops between 24 and 28 weeks of pregnancy. It is diagnosed through a routine blood test rather than by presence of symptoms. It is caused by increased levels of hormones produced by the placenta, which decrease the effectiveness of the insulin's action.

Risk factors

Gestational diabetes is more likely to develop in women who:

- are over 30
- have a previous history of gestational diabetes
- have a family history of Type 2 diabetes or pre-diabetes
- are overweight
- are indigenous Australian, from the Indian subcontinent, of Chinese or Pacific Islander background
- have a history of polycystic ovarian syndrome.

Although the diabetes usually disappears when the baby is born, approximately 50 per cent of women will go on to develop Type 2 diabetes within twenty years and as time progresses diabetes can be seen in 65 per cent of these women. The diabetes must be well managed during pregnancy and a healthy lifestyle must become a lifetime habit after the baby's birth. Medical follow up, at least two-yearly, is recommended.

Impaired fasting glucose and impaired glucose tolerance

Impaired fasting glucose (IFG) and impaired glucose tolerance (IGT) are referred to as pre-diabetes, as they can lead to the development of diabetes. These conditions affect one in six adults in Australia and can also be seen in children and adolescents.

Impaired fasting glucose is diagnosed by pathology test when the fasting blood glucose level is higher than normal but does not rise excessively after having a drink containing 75 grams pure glucose.

With Impaired glucose tolerance, the blood glucose level will rise above the normal level after drinking a 75-gram glucose drink.

Although in both cases the blood glucose levels are above normal they do not go high enough for diabetes to be diagnosed. These two conditions, also known as pre-diabetes, result from a resistance to insulin and in many cases will lead to Type 2 diabetes in later life.

Risk factors

As with Type 2 diabetes, IFG and IGT are most common in people who:

- have a family history of Type 2 diabetes
- are overweight, especially where excess weight is carried around the waistline
- are inactive.

To reduce the risk of developing Type 2 diabetes, a healthy eating pattern, regular exercise and long-term weight management is essential.

Recognising diabetes

People with one or more of the following should be tested for diabetes:

- symptoms of diabetes (see page 8)
- age over 65 for non-Indigenous Australians
- age over 35 for Indigenous Australians and other high-risk groups (including people from the Indian subcontinent, China and Pacific Islands)
- two or more risk factors (see pages 11–12).

Diagnosing diabetes

Diagnosis is made by a blood test, either fasting, random or following a special glucose drink. Fasting blood glucose is when you have been without food or drink for 10–12 hours. A random test is done anytime regardless of whether you have eaten or not. If the result is not conclusive and your doctor suspects diabetes, he or she may order an Oral Glucose Tolerance Test (OGTT) to exclude or confirm diabetes. Here, a fasting blood test is performed then 75 grams of glucose is given orally and further blood samples tested one and two hours afterwards. Tests should be repeated to confirm diagnosis.

Diagnosis	Fasting blood glucose (millimoles per litre)	Random blood glucose	OGTT Reading taken 2 hours after 75g glucose
Diabetes unlikely	<5.5 mmol/L	<5.5 mmol/L	<7.8 mmol/L
Impaired fasting glucose	6.0–6.9 mmol/L	May be normal	
Impaired glucose tolerance	May be raised		7.8–11 mmol/L
Diabetes	7.0 mmol/L or more	11.1 mmol/L or more	11.1 mmol/L or more
Gestational diabetes	>5.5 mmol/L	>7.0 mmol/L 2 hr after a meal	8.0 mmol/L or more

Note: Different laboratories and specialist centres may use figures that vary slightly from these.

Management of diabetes

Diabetes management aims to keep glucose levels close to normal. For a person without diabetes, the blood glucose level sits between approximately 3.5 and 7.8 mmol/L or millimoles per litre. This range of glucose levels is called the 'normal range'. For a person with pre-diabetes or diabetes the amount of glucose in the blood increases above the normal range.

When the blood glucose level increases above the normal range people can experience 'short term complications of diabetes'. These are the same as the symptoms of undiagnosed diabetes because the cause is the same: high blood glucose levels. The aim of managing diabetes is to keep blood glucose levels as close to normal (non-diabetic) levels as possible.

Prolonged high blood glucose levels may cause damage to the body

If the blood glucose level remains high or fluctuates excessively over a period of time this may cause damage to the body. This damage is known as the 'long term complications of diabetes' and includes damage to the blood vessels that supply your eyes, kidneys, heart and other organs and nerves.

In the longer term this can lead to problems such as:
- loss of vision
- kidney disease
- heart disease
- loss of sensation and/or intermittent pain in the extremities, particularly the legs and feet
- impaired healing and immune responses and increased risk of infection and ulcers.

Learning how to manage your diabetes and achieving good blood glucose management is the best way to avoid these complications.

Early diagnosis results in better health outcomes

The earlier diabetes is diagnosed, the earlier management strategies can be put in place. Management strategies reduce the risk of short- and long-term complications of diabetes and maximise health outcomes.

Diabetes management focuses on different approaches for different people and may involve:

- diet and exercise
- diet, exercise and diabetes tablets
- diet, exercise and insulin (by injection or insulin pump)
- diet, exercise, tablets and insulin.

The approach most beneficial for you will depend on what type of diabetes you have as well as your weight and blood glucose level.

Weight management, regular exercise, monitoring and follow up are essential

You probably understand your body and the way it reacts to treatment better than anyone else, so you should be an important part of your management team. The more you understand about how to manage your own diabetes the better your health is likely to be. Weight management, regular exercise, blood glucose monitoring and regular medical review and monitoring are essential for good management.

Weight management will help blood glucose management

If you are overweight, weight loss will help you to manage your blood glucose levels, particularly if you are carrying excess weight around your waist. The amount of weight you need to lose to optimise glucose levels is individual but improvements occur with even modest weight loss. For more information about weight management refer to page 33.

Exercise is a cornerstone of good diabetes management

Regular exercise is critical for health and wellbeing and is a cornerstone of diabetes management, especially for people with Type 2 diabetes and gestational diabetes. For those with Type 1 diabetes, the relationship between exercise and blood glucose management is more complex. Regular exercise might include walking, swimming, taking the stairs, playing bowls or tennis, going for a bike ride, Tai Chi, yoga, weightlifting or walking to the shops instead of driving. Whatever exercise you choose, and whatever level of physical activity you find most comfortable, aim to make it a regular part of your life. **Thirty minutes of exercise, 5 times a week is a good goal for most people**. If you can manage more than this it is better but if not, remember that any exercise is better than none at all.

Home monitoring of blood glucose is done using a blood glucose meter. A finger is pricked and a drop of blood placed on a test strip which is then inserted into the meter. The meter displays the glucose level in the blood. Your doctor or diabetes educator will discuss blood monitoring with you and advise you on how to test your own blood glucose levels. Ask your doctor or diabetes educator how often and when to test and how you should record the results.

For most people a target for blood glucose should be 4–6 mmol/L before meals and up to 8 mmol/L after meals.

Follow up helps ensure that your management strategies are working

Regular follow up by your doctor, dietitian and diabetes educator helps to ensure you are kept informed and that your management strategies are tailored for you and your changing needs. Show your blood glucose level records to your doctor, diabetes educator or dietitian at follow-up appointments. If you do not monitor your own blood glucose, have your doctor do this on a regular basis.

Your doctor may order a glycosylated haemoglobin (HbA1c) blood test as an indication of your long term blood glucose management. This test measures the glucose that attaches to the red blood cell and shows your average blood glucose level over the preceding 10–12 weeks. A result less than 7% is an indication of good diabetes management.

The following criterion is used to assess diabetes management:
* normal range: 4.0–6.0%
* good control: 6.1–7.0%
* fair control: 7.1–7.9%
* poor control: greater than 8.0%.

Your doctor should also check your blood pressure and order blood fat tests regularly.

It is essential to have your eyes, feet and teeth checked regularly, even if you have dentures. These regular checks are important as:
* diabetes and high blood glucose can cause fluctuations in the eye's ability to focus and lead to serious damage to the blood vessels in the eyes
* diabetes and high blood glucose can lead to nerve damage and poor blood flow in the legs and feet and a lowered ability to feel pain, heat and cold. This may result in a sore or cut on a foot which may be slow to heal
* long-term or chronic dental infection increases risk of developing blood vessel disease and heart attacks.

Follow up is important as it helps you and your management team detect and manage early signs of long-term diabetes complications.

Ask questions. Don't be shy or worry that you seem stupid or are being a bother. No matter how silly you think your question may be, ask it. Keep on asking until you are entirely satisfied that you understand your diabetes and know what to do to manage it. If, like many, you tend to go blank when seeing the dietitian, doctor or diabetes educator, sit down before your visit and write out your questions and concerns. Take your list with you and go through it item by item.

Health professionals are often busy. If you need extra time, make an appointment for a less busy time or ask for a double appointment. You can also take a family member, friend or partner to help you remember what was said and to support you if you feel anxious or unable to ask questions.

Follow the advice of your health professionals and not the advice of friends, relative or neighbours, however well-intentioned. There is much misinformation about diabetes in the community, and appropriate management differs from person to person—what suits someone else may not be right for you.

Food for health and diabetes

Food is an important part of life—it is a necessity and it should also be a pleasure. Diabetes does not need to change this. What we eat is a very individual matter. How you feel at any particular moment, your taste preferences, your cultural background and lifestyle, all have an effect on your food choices. The enjoyment we get from food should be matched by its value as a source of nourishment and its role in helping you maintain good health.

Nutrients in foods

The nutrients in food include protein, fat, carbohydrate, vitamins, minerals, fibre, phytochemicals and water. Foods provide a range of different textures, flavours, colours and nutritional value, and eating a variety will ensure you get what you need for good health.

Dietary guidelines and diabetes

A good guide for choosing a healthy diet is set out in the Dietary Guidelines for Australians. These guidelines have been developed by The National Health and Medical Research Council (NHMRC) in consultation with many experts in the area of health and nutrition. They are based on scientific evidence and are designed to prevent or minimise the development of diet-related diseases, including diabetes. The dietary guidelines encourage the intake of an eating pattern and lifestyle which promotes good nutrition and health. This is ideal for the management of a person with diabetes or pre-diabetes.

In this section, we will explain why these guidelines are important. We discuss those that are particularly important if you have diabetes, but don't ignore the rest.

Australian Dietary Guidelines

- Enjoy a wide variety of nutritious foods.
- Eat plenty of vegetables, legumes and fruits.
- Eat plenty of cereals (including breads, rice, pasta and noodles), preferably wholegrain.
- Include lean meat, fish, poultry and/or alternatives.
- Include milks, yoghurts, cheeses and/or alternatives. Reduced-fat varieties should be chosen, where possible.
- Drink plenty of water.
- Take care to:
  - limit saturated fat and moderate total fat intake
  - choose foods low in salt
  - limit your alcohol intake if you choose to drink
  - consume only moderate amounts of sugars and foods containing added sugars.
- Prevent weight gain: be physically active and eat according to your energy needs.
- Care for your food: prepare and store it safely.
- Encourage and support breastfeeding.

National Health and Medical Research Council, 2003

Dietary Guidelines: Eat plenty of vegetables, legumes, fruits and cereals (including breads, rice, pasta and noodles), preferably wholegrain

Carbohydrate

These foods should form a major part of your diet. They contain plenty of carbohydrate, which is the body's main source of energy. They also provide vitamins, minerals and phytochemicals. Eating them regularly will help you manage your diabetes. They will also help you control your weight because they are satisfying and bulky.

There are three broad groups of carbohydrates:

- sugar
- starch
- fibre.

Sugar and starch both get broken down into glucose which is absorbed from the gut into the bloodstream.

Fibre does not get broken down and absorbed into the bloodstream like sugar and starch. Fibre stays in the gut, adding bulk and absorbing water. It travels all the way down the gut and is excreted as stool (faeces). Fibre does not contribute glucose into the bloodstream.

Nutrition tip—Carbohydrate:

- sugars and starches are the most important energy sources for all body tissues, especially the brain
- plays an important part in many body functions.

You find starches in breads, biscuits, cereals, grains, some vegetables and pulses.

Sugars are found naturally in fruit, milk and honey, and are added as sweeteners to many foods such as confectionery, cakes, chocolate, soft drinks and jams. Foods high in added sugars and starches are often low in nutrients and/or may be high in saturated fat.

Vegetables

Include plenty of non-starchy vegetables in your daily diet together with starchy ones. It is recommended that you should eat at least 5 serves of vegetables daily. (½ cup = 1 serve)

Starchy vegetables include potatoes, sweet potatoes, sweetcorn, parsnips and yams.

Vegetables, other than starchy ones, are low in carbohydrate, but high in fibre, and are a particularly rich source of minerals and vitamins.

Nutrition tip—Vitamins:

- help the body use the energy from carbohydrate, fat and protein
- play an essential part in body functions, including growth and repair of body tissues.

There are two main groups of vitamins:

- water-soluble vitamins—the B group and C. These are found widely in foods including fruits, vegetables, cereals, milk and meat
- fat-soluble vitamins—A, D, E and K. These are found in animal fats such as butter, other dairy products, meat, fish, vegetable oils and margarines, wholegrain products, nuts and seeds.

Nutrition tip—Minerals:

- form major part of bones, teeth and body fluids such as blood
- play an essential part in body functions such as heart beat, muscle contraction, and in the nervous system and fluid balance
- occur widely in foods such as meat and fish, milk and cheese, fruits, vegetables and cereals.

Legumes

Legumes, also called pulses, include dried beans (such as red kidney, borlotti, black-eyed, haricot, cannellini, baked beans and soy beans), peas (such as split peas and chick peas) and lentils.

Fruit

Include all varieties, particularly fresh. It is recommended that you include at least two serves of fruit in your diet daily.

Nutrition tip—Phytochemicals:
- reduce risk of certain diseases including many cancers, cardiovascular disorders and diabetes
- are found in plant foods; rich sources include fruits, vegetables, pulses, including soybeans, herbs, tea, red and white wine, nuts and olive oil.

Bread and cereals

Include bread, breakfast cereals, rice, wheat, barley, oats, buckwheat, rye, pasta (such as spaghetti and noodles).

Both starches and sugars have the potential to increase the blood glucose level

Sugar and starch carbohydrates are broken down into glucose which is absorbed into the blood where your body uses it for energy. It is important to include adequate high carbohydrate foods in each meal, for example bread, pasta, potato, rice, milk, yoghurt or fruit. This will provide your body with the energy required for your daily activities. Approximately 50% of your total energy intake should come from these foods. If you are young and/or active, your carbohydrate requirements will be higher than older or less active people.

Sugar (sucrose or cane sugar) used to be considered as the main component in food that increased blood glucose levels. We now know that both starches and sugars have the potential to increase the blood glucose level. This is because they both contain glucose.

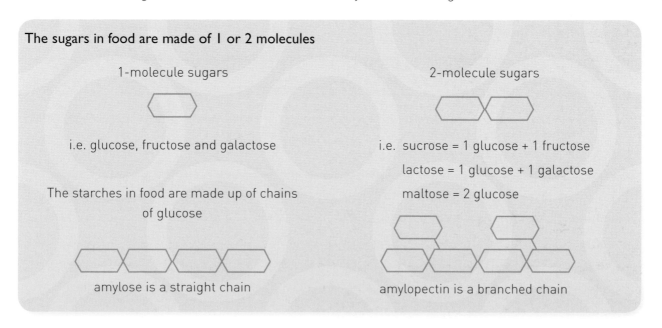

The sugars in food are made of 1 or 2 molecules

1-molecule sugars	2-molecule sugars

i.e. glucose, fructose and galactose

i.e. sucrose = 1 glucose + 1 fructose

lactose = 1 glucose + 1 galactose

maltose = 2 glucose

The starches in food are made up of chains of glucose

amylose is a straight chain

amylopectin is a branched chain

The glycaemic index

Different foods have different effects on the blood glucose level. This is because foods are broken down and/or absorbed at different rates.

Foods that are broken down and absorbed more quickly cause a quicker and higher rise in blood glucose levels than those that are broken down and absorbed more slowly.

The effect of food on blood glucose levels is measured by the glycaemic index (GI). This is how it works:

- Carbohydrate-containing foods are rated 1 to 100 according to their impact on the blood glucose level.
- Foods that cause a smaller rise in the blood glucose have a lower GI number.
- Foods that cause a greater rise have a higher GI number.
- Good management of diabetes is helped by regularly eating foods with a low GI number.

Pure glucose has a glycaemic index of 100

The GI of a food is calculated by measuring what happens to a person's blood glucose level after the food is eaten. An amount of the food containing 50 grams of carbohydrate is eaten and the person's blood glucose level is tested at intervals over a 2-hour period. The blood glucose level is graphed to show how quickly and to what extent the food made the glucose levels rise.

Pure glucose is absorbed into the blood stream more quickly than other carbohydrates. It produces a graph with the largest rise and is given a GI rating of 100. Other foods have smaller rises and have GI's less than 100.

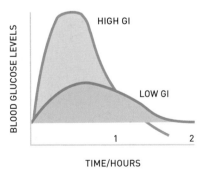

Factors affecting the GI of foods

- amount of processing
- preparation and cooking
- type of sugar or starch
- amount and type of fibre
- acidity of the food
- amount of fat present in the food.

Fat slows digestion and lowers the GI rating of foods but a high fat diet is generally not recommended because excessive fat in the diet can lead to weight gain and high blood fats. For more information about fats in the diet refer to page 26.

Lower GI foods help the management of blood glucose levels

Include foods of lower GI regularly in your diet to help manage blood glucose levels. It is recommended that **at least one lower GI food (as listed below) is included at each meal**. For those who eat between meals, it is best to choose lower GI snacks.

The foods that are lower in GI include:

- pulses/legumes (all varieties)
- porridge, Allbran™ and rice bran
- breads containing large amounts of wholegrains such as pumpernickel, wholegrain rye and wheat, soy and linseed, oats and barley, genuine sour dough, white breads displaying the GI symbol
- barley, buckwheat, bulgar
- all wheat-based pastas (including spaghetti) and fresh rice noodles
- fruits from temperate climates such as apples, grapes, grapefruit, oranges, peaches, pears, plums and firm bananas
- some vegetables such as sweet potatoes, yam and sweetcorn
- some rice such as Mahatma™ long-grain white rice, basmati and doongara (an Australian variety), fresh rice noodles, sushi where rice is acidic (as it is cooked in rice vinegar).
- fat-reduced milk and yoghurt.

Foods with a high GI may be eaten regularly

Many foods with a high GI provide important nutrients and variety so they can be eaten as part of a healthy eating pattern. When you eat high GI foods it is important to combine them with low GI ones to help level out the rise in blood glucose levels. It is also best to keep serving sizes of high GI foods small. Your dietitian will help you balance these foods to suit your food preferences and lifestyle.

Carbohydrate-rich foods can be classified as high, medium or low GI

By using the Glycaemic Index rating, carbohydrate-rich foods can be classified as:

- high GI—index number of 70 or more
- medium GI—index number 56–69
- low GI—index number of 55 or less.

This information is current, but research continues and there may be further changes in the future.

The food value lists at the end of this book show the Glycaemic Index of many foods, along with carbohydrate, fat and energy levels. These may be used as a guide to food choice.

Fibre

The Dietary Guideline encouraging us to eat plenty of vegetables, legumes, fruits and cereals is important as these foods provide us with our dietary fibre.

Eating plenty of foods that are high in fibre and lower in GI will help you manage your blood glucose levels, satisfy your appetite and promote heart and bowel health. Achieve this by:

- choosing wholegrain breakfast cereals, especially those high in bran or rolled oats
- choosing heavy wholegrain or sourdough bread, or wholemeal and white breads that are promoted as low GI
- using plenty of legumes in cooking, including baked beans, lentils, kidney beans, cannelloni beans and chickpeas. Add to soups, casseroles, salads, savoury dishes and dips. The tinned varieties can be used for convenience.
- eating at least 5 serves of vegetables every day and trying to have as much variety as possible. Serve vegetables cooked or in salads and include in soups, sauces and meat dishes
- eating at least two pieces of fruit daily. Preferably eat them fresh rather than cooked, and don't drink more than one small glass of fruit or vegetable juice per day, as this is low in fibre
- leaving vegetables and fruit unpeeled, where possible, for maximum fibre.

Nutrition tip—Fibre:

- has several tasks, including keeping the digestive tract in good shape. In other words, it keeps our bowels functioning regularly and easily
- helps fill the stomach, satisfies our appetite and helps to limit overeating
- some types of fibre, particularly oats and psyllium husks, help remove the cholesterol from the gut before it gets into the blood
- is invaluable in your diet. Eat lots of it. Good sources of fibre include wholegrain breads and cereals, fruits, vegetables and pulses.

Dietary Guideline: Consume only moderate amounts of sugars and foods containing added sugars

Added sugars

Many processed foods contain added sugars. You will find sugar in many forms, some obvious, some less so, in many of the foods you buy. High-sugar foods are high in kilojoules (calories) but often low in other nutrients. This means they can add to your energy intake without providing any useful nourishment. High-sugar foods are also often high in fat for instance, cakes, sweet biscuits and chocolate.

As sugar has a medium GI rating, you can eat small amounts of sugar without making your blood glucose levels rise excessively. For instance, using a moderate amount of jam on wholegrain toast or adding a teaspoon of sugar to a bowl of porridge.

Eating too much sugar is not a good idea as it adds to your total kilojoule (calorie) intake without providing any vitamins, minerals or other beneficial nutrients. You can train your palate to enjoy foods with far less sugar than we have become accustomed to in our Western diet.

Hints to help you cut down on sugar

- Check product labels. Read the section 'making sense of food labels' (page 62).
- Water is the best thirst quencher. If you must drink soft drinks, have low-joule (low-calorie) ones, flavoured mineral waters and cordials instead of the regular varieties.
- Avoid sugar in tea, coffee or other beverages.
- Replace processed snack foods with fresh fruit, nuts, yoghurt, a slice of wholegrain or sourdough bread, toast with topping, or chopped raw vegetables (such as carrot, celery, tomato or capsicum).
- Buy solid pack unsweetened canned fruit, fruit packed in water or natural juice, or artificially sweetened canned fruit instead of fruit canned in syrups.
- If you want flavoured jellies, use the low-joule (low-calorie) products.
- Look for recipes with small to moderate amounts of sugar, fructose or honey. Our recipes will give you a guide to just how little sugar or sweetness you need to add to make food delicious.
- Low-fat fruit yoghurts are often surprisingly high in sugar. Choose those that are artificially sweetened or make your own by combining low-fat natural yoghurt and your choice of fresh or stewed fruits.

Dietary Guideline: Drink plenty of water

Water

A good fluid intake is important for health and wellbeing. Although there are plenty of different drinks that you can have, plain water is good as it provides no additional kilojoules (calories).

Nutrition tip—Water:

- is an essential part of every body function—about two-thirds of the body is water
- is the best drink for health. Don't wait until you're thirsty. Unless your doctor advises you otherwise, drink at least six to eight cups of fluid a day, and you will feel the benefit.

Dietary Guideline: Limit saturated fat and moderate total fat intake.

Fats

Fat is a taste-enhancer and adds texture to foods. It also provides fat-soluble vitamins and essential fatty acids. Unfortunately, many of us have become used to eating too much of it. Fat is the most concentrated form of energy we eat, providing more than twice the amount of kilojoules (calories) per gram than both carbohydrate and protein. Not only do we use it knowingly by frying foods or by ladling on the cream, but also by eating too many processed foods.

We eat a great deal of fat in processed foods. It is sobering to realise that:

- a 100-gram packet of potato crisps contains 40% fat and 2385 kilojoules (570 calories), which is roughly quarter of the average daily energy requirements
- a plain unsweetened shop-bought biscuit may have as much as 20% fat and 262 kilojoules (63 calories).

Generally a moderate fat intake is recommended. A diet high in fat can lead to excessive weight gain, which in turn can increase insulin resistance by inhibiting insulin activity. A diet high in fat is often unbalanced because foods that are high in fat can displace more nutritious low fat foods such as fruit, vegetables and wholegrain cereals.

Nutrition tip—Fat:

- provides a concentrated form of energy
- plays an important part in insulating and protecting the body's organs and other tissues
- transports other nutrients into and around the body.

Only small amounts of fat are needed to perform these important tasks.

Major sources include butter, margarine, oils, meats and poultry, cheese, fried and takeaway foods, dips, potato crisps, nuts, seeds, snack foods, cream, dressings, cakes, biscuits, pastries and chocolate.

On the other hand, a diet that is too low in fat may be overly restrictive, boring and less satisfying. It can also lead to a deficiency in fat soluble vitamins and the essential fatty acids, omega 3 and omega 6 fats, which the body is unable to make. A moderate fat intake will provide plenty of these essential nutrients.

Choose foods that are low in saturated fat

Saturated fats increase the risk of heart disease by increasing cholesterol levels which narrow blood vessels and contribute to blocking of these.

Choose foods that are low in saturated fat. Saturated fats are the fats found in:
- animal products, such as butter, lard, ghee, dripping, meat fats, cream and cheese
- commercially baked goods, such as biscuits and pastries
- two plant products, palm oil and coconut fat (e.g.copha, coconut milk and coconut cream).

See page 62 for the different ways in which saturated fat can be identified in an ingredients list.

Replacing saturated with monounsaturated fats can improve insulin sensitivity

Studies have shown that replacing saturated fats with monounsaturated ones can improve insulin sensitivity although this will not increase the amount of insulin your body makes. This effect is only seen in people who have a low to moderate fat intake and not in those who have a high fat diet. Read labels where possible and limit the use of commercially prepared high-fat and fried foods.

Eat moderate amounts of polyunsaturated and monounsaturated fats

Polyunsaturated and monounsaturated fats are generally the fats found in fish and plant foods. They include the fats and oils in:
- oily fish such as mackerel, salmon, herrings and sardines
- polyunsaturated and monounsaturated margarines
- sunflower, safflower, olive, canola and peanut oils
- avocado, nuts, seeds and olives.

Eat moderate amounts of polyunsaturated and monounsaturated fats. Compared to saturated fat they are the healthy option for spreads and in cooking and dressings. Polyunsaturated and monounsaturated fats add flavour and nutrients to the diet and can make meals more satisfying. They will not increase cholesterol levels but if taken in excess may lead to weight gain.

All fats, whether saturated or unsaturated, provide the same amount of kilojoules (calories) per gram. Large amounts can lead to weight gain. Carrying excess weight can increase blood glucose and blood cholesterol levels.

Cholesterol

Cholesterol is a fatty substance which can be made in the liver or obtained from food we eat. It is essential for life and:
- forms part of cell walls
- is the basis of many hormones
- is used to make Vitamin D
- forms the basis of bile which helps us digest fats.

Fats and heart disease

- The different types of fats in foods are important as they have different effects on blood fat levels and heart disease.
- The main fats in foods are saturated, monounsaturated or polyunsaturated according to their different structures. These fats can be found in both animal and plant foods.
- **Cholesterol** is also a type of fat present in food and made in the body. It is only found in animal foods.
- Although eating too much cholesterol may increase the cholesterol level in your blood, saturated fats have a much greater effect.
- Some processed foods contain vegetable oils which have been converted to either saturated or trans fats. **Trans fat** has a similar effect in the body to saturated fat. Eating too much saturated and trans fats (and cholesterol) may cause the fats to rise in the blood and high blood fats can lead to heart and blood vessel disease.

Fats found in fish are rich in the polyunsaturated fats called omega 3 fats. Omega 3 fats need to be in the food we eat as they cannot be made in the body. They are important for health as they help reduce blood pressure and blood clotting, help keep the blood vessels flexible, help maintain a steady heart rhythm and reduce inflammation.

In the body there is good cholesterol (known as high density lipoprotein cholesterol or HDL-C) and bad cholesterol (known as low density lipoprotein cholesterol or LDL-C). Good cholesterol helps prevent the bad cholesterol being deposited on the blood vessel walls whilst the bad cholesterol can be deposited inside the blood vessels in a substance known as 'plaque'. This causes a narrowing or 'hardening' of the arteries and restricts blood flow. At times, pieces of plaque can lead to blockages in the blood vessels of the heart causing a heart attack.

Using fat in a healthy way

- Eat less processed, takeaway and convenience foods.
- Order a side salad or vegetables instead of chips when eating out.
- Many dry/savoury biscuits are high in fat: eat these occasionally or use low fat options or bread, toast or pita.
- Select small serves of lean meats or poultry; trim off excess fat and skin (see page 179).
- Use margarine, avocado or peanut butter in preference to butter.
- Use low-fat dairy products to help keep your intake of saturated fat low.
- Grill or bake meat on a rack to allow fat to drain away.
- If you like sour cream as a dressing on vegetable or meat dishes, use a natural yoghurt or low-fat ricotta or cottage cheese, or try some of our low fat dips instead.

Understanding fats

Saturated fats	Trans fats
Dairy fats: cheese, cream, sour cream, butter Meat fat, processed meats, chicken skin Lard, ghee, dripping, tallow Coconut milk and cream Frize and other hard cooking fats Palm oil: found in many commercial foods (snack foods, takeaways and baked goodssuch as pastry, cakes, biscuits	Butter, milk fat, beef and lamb Hard margarines Solidified fats and some margarines used in commercial baking and pastry making

Unsaturated fats can be polyunsaturated or monounsaturated. Polyunsaturated fats provide the essential fatty acids, omega 6 and omega 3.

Polyunsaturated fats		Monounsaturated fats
Omega 6 Sunflower oil Corn oil Soybean oil Safflower oil Sesame oil Grapeseed oil Ricebran	**Omega 3** Fish oil Oily fish Flaxseed/linseed Canola oil Nuts (walnut, pecan) Very lean meat oatbran	Olive oil Canola oil Avocado Sunola oil Nuts (peanut, macadamia, cashew, almond, pistachio and pecan)

- Use low fat custard or yoghurt, or a small amount of ice-cream instead of cream on desserts.
- Save cream and sour cream for special occasions only and then use them in small amounts.
- Aim to eat two to three serves of fish per week (include oily fish where possible, for example salmon, mackerel, sardines and herring) (see page 168).
- Learn to use fresh or dried herbs, spices, onion, tomato or lemon juice to add flavour to food instead of just relying on fat and salt.
- Use moderate amounts of oil in cooking and choose poly- or mono-unsaturated oils.

High blood fat levels, poor sleep patterns and smoking increase cardiovascular risk

People who have diabetes and/or high blood fat levels have an increased risk of heart and blood vessel disease. The blood fats of concern are cholesterol and triglycerides. Both of these fats are made in the body as well as being provided in foods. High triglyceride levels may also be found in overweight people and in people with undiagnosed or poorly managed diabetes. Weight loss, a low-fat eating pattern and establishing good management of diabetes will help reduce these levels. It is strongly recommended that smokers, unable to stop by themselves, seek help to break the habit.

Poor sleep patterns or sleep apnoea can increase your risk of developing cardiovascular disease as can infections caused by poor dental health. If you have these problems, discuss them with your doctor.

Limit saturated fats in your diet. If you are concerned about the amount of fat in your diet or require greater detail on the types of fats, consult a dietitian or your state division of The Heart Foundation www.heartfoundation.org.au.

Dietary Guidelines: Include lean meat, fish, poultry, milk, yoghurt, cheeses and/or alternatives.

Protein

Protein is important to a healthy eating plan and you should include some every day. You only need one or two small serves of protein daily. Protein rich foods often contain fat, so be aware of this when you make choices.

Nutrition tip—Protein:
- is an important part of all body tissues, enzymes, hormones and the immune system
- is required for body growth and repair
- the richest sources are meat, poultry, fish, seafood, eggs, milk products, tofu, pulses, nuts and seeds

Meat, poultry and fish

- Meat and poultry provide many essential nutrients as well as protein. These include vitamins B, iron and zinc, although poultry is not as rich in iron or zinc as red meat.
- When choosing these foods, select those which are lower in fat, such as lean beef, veal, pork or lamb; fish and seafood; chicken or turkey without skin; lean game meat such as rabbit, buffalo, venison and kangaroo.
- To be classified as lean, meat should have minimal visible fat marbled through it, and you should trim off any fat around the meat before you cook it.
- Eat less high fat meats such as sausages, salami and processed meats.
- One serve meat or fish = 80–125 grams of raw lean. For most people, a piece of cooked meat or fish the size of the palm of their hand will be adequate.
- Include 2–3 serves of fish per week. Oily fish, which includes most of the types of fish available in cans, are good as they are high in omega 3 fats.

Eggs

- Eggs are low in fat and, although the yolk is rich in cholesterol, current research shows this has little effect on blood cholesterol level in most people.
- Two eggs make a good serve and an intake of up to 6 eggs per week is fine unless advised otherwise by your doctor or dietitian.

Milk and milk products

- Regular milk and yoghurt can be high in fat and contain predominantly saturated fats. Choose low fat varieties.
- Milk and yoghurt contain the carbohydrate lactose (milk sugar).
- One cup of milk or yoghurt will give you roughly the same amount of carbohydrate as a slice of bread.
- Cheese is high in fat, even many fat reduced cheeses are high in fat. Use cheese as an 'occasional' food. If you eat a lot of cheese, try to replace it where there are alternatives. For example, replace cheese in a sandwich with avocado, lean meat, egg or smoked salmon.

Tofu (soybean curd)

- Tofu is low in fat and rich in protein and B-vitamins.
- It is bland to taste but readily absorbs the flavour of other foods during cooking.
- The consistency of tofu can vary and is described as being firm, soft or silken: firm tofu is dense and can be cubed and added to stir-fries and soups; soft tofu tends to fall apart more easily and is good for blending; silken tofu is soft and creamy and can be used to replace cream or sour cream in savoury recipes and in dips.

Pulses (legumes)

- These include dried peas, beans and lentils.
- Pulses are excellent as a source of protein and have the added advantage of being low in fat.
- They make an ideal alternative or addition to meat dishes.
- They are rich in carbohydrate and have a lower GI.
- Pulses provide iron and fibre and useful amounts of calcium, potassium and B vitamins.
- Three-quarters of a cup of cooked pulses is a good serve size.

Nuts and seeds

- Nuts and seeds and products made from them, such as peanut butter and tahini, are a valuable source of protein, but are high in unsaturated fats and kilojoules (calories).
- If overweight, only eat nuts and seeds in small amounts.

A special note on milk

Dairy products are important sources of protein and calcium. Calcium plays a vital part in good bone health and helps protect from osteoporosis (loss of calcium from bones, making them brittle).

- Adult men should include at least 2 serves of dairy products daily.
- Children, adolescents, adult women (including those who are pregnant, breastfeeding or post-menopausal) and men over 70 years should include at least 3 serves of dairy products daily.
  * 1 serve = 250ml milk (1 cup), 200g (6½oz) yoghurt, 40g piece of cheese

Dietary Guideline: Limit your alcohol intake if you choose to drink.

Alcohol

Alcoholic drinks are high in kilojoules (calories) and can contribute to weight gain.

If you drink alcohol, drink it with food, in moderation and with good sense. Recent research has indicated that 1 or 2 standard drinks a day may offer some health benefits and help insulin work better. Any benefits are lost if more than this is drunk. Excessive alcohol consumption is significantly harmful to health and may make diabetes more difficult to manage. It is recommended that you avoid drinking any alcohol for two days each week.

Nutrition tip—Alcohol:

- is not a nutrient
- provides concentrated energy, but it isn't usually considered a nutrient
- components, including phytochemicals, may offer health protection.

Adults should limit alcohol intake to two or less standard drinks in any one day

The National Health and Medical Research Council's (NHMRC) '2009 Australian Guidelines to Reduce Health Risks from Drinking Alcohol' recommends adult males and females should limit alcohol intake to two standard drinks or less a day. See www.nhmrc.gov.au/publications. Intakes greater than these may have adverse effects on health and may make diabetes difficult to manage.

Read the labels on the bottles and cans as the alcohol content, particularly of wine and beer, can vary greatly between products.

Most diet beers contain the same alcohol as regular beer

'Diabetic' or 'diet' beers are lower in carbohydrate but contain as much alcohol and kilojoules as regular beers. Low alcohol (less than 3% alcohol) beers are recommended over regular beers.

Guide to standard drinks

(approximately 10g alcohol)

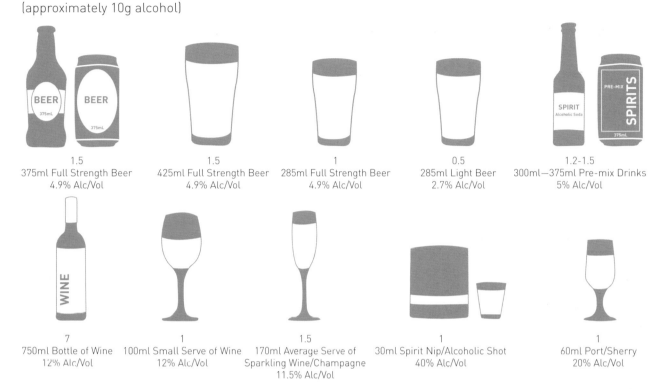

1.5	1.5	1	0.5	1.2-1.5
375ml Full Strength Beer 4.9% Alc/Vol	425ml Full Strength Beer 4.9% Alc/Vol	285ml Full Strength Beer 4.9% Alc/Vol	285ml Light Beer 2.7% Alc/Vol	300ml—375ml Pre-mix Drinks 5% Alc/Vol

7	1	1.5	1	1
750ml Bottle of Wine 12% Alc/Vol	100ml Small Serve of Wine 12% Alc/Vol	170ml Average Serve of Sparkling Wine/Champagne 11.5% Alc/Vol	30ml Spirit Nip/Alcoholic Shot 40% Alc/Vol	60ml Port/Sherry 20% Alc/Vol

Rather than a regular mixer, a low-joule soft drink, soda water or plain mineral water mixed with spirits will help lower kilojoule (calorie) and sugar intake if you are watching your weight.

Alcohol may react with medication and lead to a drop in blood glucose level

If you are taking hypoglycaemic medication and you drink alcohol without having carbohydrate, the alcohol may react with your medication and your blood glucose levels may drop too low. This may lead to hypoglycaemia (low blood glucose). Don't drink alcohol on an empty stomach. Always eat some starchy food when you drink, for example, a dry biscuit or a meal which includes carbohydrate with your wine. Fruit juice and milk contain carbohydrate.

Dietary Guideline: Prevent weight gain: be physically active and eat according to your energy needs

Weight management

Being overweight makes diabetes more difficult to manage. The extra body fat makes it more difficult for the insulin to carry the glucose into the cells and as a result, the blood glucose levels remain too high. This is particularly the case with excess weight around the abdomen. Even modest weight loss (for example 5% of body weight) can help insulin work more effectively again.

> **Fat stored around the central body increases the risk of diabetes**
>
> Women of childbearing age tend to store their fat in the lower part of the body (pear-shape) whilst men and postmenopausal women tend to store it around the central body; the waist and abdomen (apple-shape). With excessive weight gain, fat is stored around the central body. This increases the risk to health generally and increases the chance of developing diabetes and cardiovascular disease.
>
> Pears are healthier than apples … so measure your waist.
>
> If you are of Caucasian origin, a waist measurement greater than 80 centimetres for women and 90 centimetres for men increases the risk of developing Type 2 diabetes.

If you are overweight, losing weight helps diabetes management

If you are overweight, losing weight is the key to good diabetes management, and should be a priority. It will also benefit your overall health. Whether you need to maintain or lose weight, the guidelines given in this book will help you achieve your goal.

Lose weight by reducing kilojoule (calorie) and fat intake

Put simply, weight loss is promoted by reducing total kilojoule (calorie) intake and increasing physical activity. While you are losing weight, it is important to maintain your health by eating regular meals that supply all your nutritional needs. Avoid crash diets and quick solutions—they offer no long-term benefits. Developing a healthy eating pattern over a long period of time will help you to achieve and maintain a lower weight. A dietitian can help you plan an eating pattern to suit your individual needs and food preferences.

Dietary Guideline: Choose foods low in salt.

Salt

Many Australians eat too much salt: in the foods they buy, in what they add in cooking and in the salt they sprinkle on their food. A high salt intake is associated with several health conditions, including fluid retention and high blood pressure and increases the risk of heart attacks and strokes. Avoiding an excess of salt is of particular importance for people with diabetes where the risk of cardiovascular and kidney problems is increased.

Limit intake of processed foods and cut back on added salt

Cut back on your salt intake by:
- limiting the amount of processed and takeaway food you eat
- limiting the amount of salt you use in cooking
- avoiding adding salt at the table.

Here is a list of some of the flavouring agents and processed foods that are high in salt:

- rock, flavoured and vegetable salts—all of them are salt, no matter what the name
- monosodium glutamate (MSG or flavour enhancer 621), flavour boosters, meat and vegetable extracts, broth, stock cubes, stock powders and packet soups
- salted, smoked, cured or pickled meat and fish
- condiments (sauces), pickles, chutneys, relishes and dressings
- canned meat, fish and vegetables
- salted snacks, including potato and corn crisps, nuts and salted biscuits
- takeaway foods such as pizza and barbecued chicken
- cheese.

Salt substitutes replace all or part of the sodium chloride with potassium chloride. These may be used to replace ordinary salt, but it is usually recommended that you to train your taste buds to enjoy low-salt foods. Always check with your doctor before using these substitutes, especially if you have kidney or heart problems.

There are many commercial products that are salt-reduced, such as breads, biscuits, margarines, butters, sauces, canned fish and vegetables. Use them in place of the regular products and learn to read labels. Look out for the words sodium and salt and for the food additive number 621 as this stands for monosodium glutamate.

Add zest to your food without adding salt by using herbs and spices. Try adding lemon juice, tomato, onion, garlic or vinegar for extra flavour.

High blood pressure may be helped by cutting back on salt

Many people with high blood pressure can bring it down by limiting the amount of salt in their diet. If overweight, also try to reduce your weight and maintain a regular exercise pattern as another means of managing your blood pressure.

Remember, in your quest for better health:

- eat regular meals each day

- include plenty of wholegrain bread, cereals, pulses, vegetables and fruit every day

- cut down on fats, concentrated sugars, alcohol and salt

- reduce your weight if you are overweight; if you are a healthy weight, keep it that way

- eating should be a pleasure; make sure your meals have plenty of flavour and texture

- quit smoking

- exercise regularly

- ask your doctor to check your blood pressure, blood fat and blood glucose levels regularly

- have eyes, teeth and feet checked regularly. Tell your health professional that you have diabetes.

Medication for diabetes

If you're on insulin or diabetes tablets, then you need to ask what type, its action and when to take it. These questions are best answered in conjunction with your doctor, diabetes educator and/or dietitian. Find out how to organise your medications and eating habits to complement each other. When on medication for diabetes, you may find that leaving long gaps between meals, or not eating enough carbohydrate at a meal, may cause your blood glucose level to drop too low (we discuss low blood glucose, hypoglycaemia, on page 40).

Tablets

Diabetes tablets lower your blood glucose level. There are several different types of diabetes tablets (oral hypoglycaemic agents) used in Australia. They vary in function and help lower your blood glucose level by:

- stimulating the pancreas to release more insulin
- encouraging your own insulin to work more effectively
- inhibiting the release of glucose by the liver
- slowing digestion and absorption of glucose from the gut.

Insulin

Different types of insulin, used in Australia, may be classified by when their activity starts, peaks and for how long their activity lasts. They include:

- ultra-short acting
- short acting
- immediate acting
- long acting
- pre-mixed insulin.

Your doctor will decide which insulin or combination of insulin is best for you and your lifestyle. The time you eat your carbohydrate should match the activity of your insulin. Discuss this with your doctor, diabetes educator and dietitian.

Using rapid-onset or short-acting insulin allows more flexibility in food choice

It is common for people with Type 1 diabetes to have an injection of rapid-onset or short-acting insulin, given according to blood glucose level, with each meal. This reflects the body's normal response to eating meals, where insulin levels in the blood increase as sugar from food is absorbed into the bloodstream. This allows greater flexibility in food choice as insulin dose can be adjusted to suit appetite and meal choice. Longer acting insulin is given prior to bed and helps in the management of blood glucose levels overnight.

Changes to insulin management are likely to occur in the future

Presently insulin is given by injection or an insulin pump (which delivers individually regulated amounts of insulin into the bloodstream as needed). If it was taken by mouth, it would be digested before it could be absorbed. Changes to insulin management are presently under trial and may grow in popularity in a limited number of people with Type 1 diabetes. These include:

- taking insulin by nasal spray or by mouth
- DAFNE (dose adjustment for normal eating) where people are trained to manage their own insulin regimens to allow a 'normal' dietary pattern to be followed. (Contact your State or Territory organisation of Diabetes Australia for further information.)
- pancreatic cell transplants.

Illness and diabetes

Everyone becomes ill every once in a while but when you have diabetes a common cold or other infection may cause a rise in your blood glucose level. It is important to:

- check your blood glucose levels, if you normally do so, every 2–4 hours. This will help you manage your diabetes more effectively. Those with Type 1 diabetes should also check for presence of ketones in the blood or urine
- drink plenty of fluids throughout the day
- chose foods you find easy to manage, if you are able to eat
- make sure someone knows you are ill so they are able to check up on you regularly
- contact your doctor if you are unable to check your blood glucose levels or drink adequately.

If you are not on medication, don't worry if you can't eat properly for a day or two

Contact your doctor if you:

- take tablets for your diabetes and are unable to eat
- are on insulin and unable to give your injection
- are vomiting or have diarrhoea for more than 12 hours
- feel excessively tired
- are ill for more than two days or taking longer than you would expect to feel better
- cannot check your blood glucose level regularly
- have a blood glucose consistently higher than 15 mmol/L for longer than 12 hours
- show ketones in your blood or urine
- are concerned about your health.

If your diabetes is managed without medication, don't worry if you are unable to eat properly for a day or two. Drink plenty of fluids and eat what you tolerate best. If you are unwell for longer than this, discuss it with your doctor.

If you are on medication for diabetes, keep on taking your medications and carbohydrate

If you are on insulin or diabetes tablets, you must continue with your medication as usual, no matter how awful you are feeling, and remember your insulin may need adjusting. One of the side effects of various illnesses, including the common cold, is that your blood glucose level rises, so your medications are absolutely vital to manage this. Equally importantly, you must keep on taking carbohydrate even if you are off your food. To do this, try light meals, drinks high in carbohydrate or high-carbohydrate snacks. You may find it easier to have a snack or drink every hour, rather than attempt your usual daily meal pattern. If taking insulin, check your urine or blood for ketones as presence of these can lead to vomiting and dehydration.

Try carbohydrate foods that are easily digested

The following are easy sources of carbohydrate if you are on medication:

- homemade or canned soup with toast or dry biscuits
- plain boiled rice or noodles
- mashed potato
- toast or a sandwich
- dry biscuits plain or with thinly sliced cheese, tomato or Vegemite (Promite, Marmite)
- regular lemonade, dry ginger or other soft drink or cordial
- regular commercially prepared jelly
- junket
- yoghurt

- custard
- creamy rice
- plain sweet biscuit or cake
- stewed or canned fruit
- ice-cream
- milk drinks such as egg flips or Aktavite™ or Milo™
- fruit juice
- black or white tea with sugar
- sports drink such as Gatorade™.

If nauseous or vomiting, try sipping drinks such as regular dry ginger ale or lemonade, Gastrolyte™, Lucozade™, Staminade™, Enos™, Dexsal™, dry ginger ale or lemonade mixed with ice-cream or milk. Once you can tolerate any of these, nibble on a dry biscuit or toast, sip chicken noodle soup or try grated apple mixed with a little orange juice.

Vomiting or diarrhoea

If you are vomiting or suffering from diarrhoea, be aware that it can lead to dehydration and poorly managed diabetes.

Hypoglycaemia

When your blood glucose level drops too low, this is known as 'hypoglycaemia', 'hypo' or 'insulin reaction'. Hypoglycaemia occurs when the blood glucose level drops below 4 mmol/L although this can vary in individuals. It can happen to you if you are on insulin or some diabetes tablets. It does not happen if you are managing your diabetes by diet alone.

Hypoglycaemia occurs when there is too much insulin or insufficient carbohydrate

Hypoglycaemia can occur if you:
- take too much insulin or diabetes tablets
- delay a meal too long
- don't include enough carbohydrate in your food
- do extra activity (without having extra carbohydrate foods to supply the extra energy—exercise uses your blood glucose supplies)
- drink too much alcohol or drink alcohol without carbohydrate.

Symptoms of hypoglycaemia can occur quickly

The symptoms set in quickly. You may experience one or more of the following:

- headache
- light headedness
- dizziness, vagueness, lack of concentration
- extreme hunger
- blurred vision
- sweating
- numbness or pins and needles around the mouth and fingers
- weakness, paleness, trembling, shaking
- drowsiness
- behaviour changes, or mood swings (such as bad temper, tearful, crying, aggressiveness).

These signs tell you that your blood glucose level may have dropped too low. Some people who test their blood glucose level regularly may find that their level drops too low without experiencing any symptoms. If your blood glucose level drops below 4 mmol/L it should be treated as hypoglycaemia whether you have symptoms or not.

If you have hypoglycaemia immediately eat some easily absorbed carbohydrate

1. Take some easily eaten, easily absorbed carbohydrate (high GI) to raise your blood glucose level. A pure form of glucose is best, otherwise try:

- glucose-enriched jelly beans (6–7 lollies)—available at a pharmacy or Diabetes Australia
- glucose tablets e.g. Gluc-eur™ (15g) or powder e.g. Glucodin™ (3 teaspoons) or gel e.g. Glutose™ 15 (1 tube, 15g glucose)
- Lucozade™ (½ small bottle or 1 glass).

If this is not available any form of easily absorbed carbohydrate will do:

- confectionery such as regular jelly beans, jubes and life savers™ (4–7 lollies)
- a regular (not diet) soft drink
- sugar in water (3 teaspoons in 1 cup of water)
- honey or jam (1 tablespoon).

Note: Do not use low-joule (low-calorie) soft drinks to treat hypoglycaemia. Hard lollies are suitable but more difficult to eat quickly.

2. Wait, if the symptoms don't improve in 10–15 minutes, or become worse, take more easily absorbed carbohydrate as above. Alternatively, if you are able to test your blood glucose level and still find it less than 4 mmol/L, repeat Step 1.

3. Once symptoms improve or your blood glucose levels are greater than 4 mmol/L eat some slowly absorbed carbohydrate (low GI) to prevent your blood glucose level from falling again. If your next meal is more than 20 minutes away, have a snack such as:
- a piece of fruit
- a slice of bread
- a small tub of low-fat yoghurt
- 6 small dry biscuits
- 2–3 pieces of dried fruit, e.g. apricots or figs.

Do not count any extra food taken to treat hypoglycaemia as part of your regular meal plan. Continue with your usual meals.

If not treated promptly hypoglycaemia can worsen

If not treated promptly and properly, hypoglycaemia can worsen and lead to unconsciousness. If this happens, others (family, friends, workmates) need to know the following guidelines:
- Never give an unconscious person anything to eat or drink.
- Roll the person onto their side, make sure the airway is clear, tilt the chin up and check the tongue hasn't rolled back.
- Give an injection of Glucagon if available and you are trained to give it.
- Call an ambulance immediately (dial 000) stating a 'diabetes emergency'.
- Wait with the person until the ambulance arrives.
- Once conscious the person will require carbohydrate to maintain their blood glucose level.

Medical treatment may include an injection of a hormone or a special glucose solution

Glucagon is a hormone that stimulates the liver to release glucose into the bloodstream to raise the blood glucose level. It is injected in a similar way to insulin. Your doctor or diabetes educator may recommend you have Glucagon on hand in case of a severe 'hypo' and will show you, your family and friends how to use it.

Carry a card containing information on hypoglycaemia

It is advisable to carry a small card containing the above information to assist others should you suffer a 'hypo' and become unconscious.

After you have had a hypo:

- Check your food intake to make sure you are having enough carbohydrate with each meal. If meals are delayed, have some carbohydrate in the form of a snack to tide you over.
- Check your dose of insulin or tablets carefully. Taking too much can make your blood glucose level fall too low.
- If you are more active than usual, you may need extra carbohydrate before, during and after the activity (see 'exercise, sport and diabetes', page 53).
- If you are drinking alcohol, make sure you eat food containing carbohydrate with it.

Important: If you are having 'hypos' often, consult your doctor to discuss possible causes and solutions. If your diabetes is well managed, you shouldn't have frequent 'hypos'.

Diabetes and coeliac disease

Coeliac disease is an autoimmune disease affecting the small bowel. The body produces antibodies that damage its own tissues, particularly the tissues in the small bowel, when exposed to gluten, a protein in some grains. This leads to poor absorption of nutrients. It is estimated that approximately 1 in 100 Australians will develop coeliac disease although around 80% of cases are never diagnosed.

Seek help

It is important that you learn about the sources of gluten as ingredients containing it are in many foods.

Seek help by joining the coeliac society in your state. They will provide you with invaluable information and support. Visit www.coeliac.org.au

Many of the recipes in this book are gluten free but we recommend that you also seek the help of a dietitian who can advise you on your individual needs.

Around 10% of children and adolescents with Type 1 diabetes will develop coeliac disease

Coeliac disease can also be associated with other autoimmune conditions such as Type 1 diabetes. Around 10% of children and adolescents with Type 1 diabetes will develop coeliac disease. The diabetes diagnosis is usually made first and the coeliac disease diagnosed later on routine screening. Although it is often suspected that coeliac disease may have been present before the diagnosis of diabetes, there may be no obvious symptoms.

Type 2 diabetes can also develop in people with coeliac disease or coeliac disease can also be diagnosed in persons with Type 2 diabetes.

Symptoms vary greatly in severity and some people show no symptoms

Coeliac disease can be diagnosed at any age and the symptoms can vary in severity. Symptoms may start in young infants when solids are first introduced. Others may be diagnosed as children, adolescents or adults and many may never be diagnosed

The treatment of coeliac diesease is life-long avoidance of gluten

People with coeliac disease are unable to tolerate cereal products containing gluten. The treatment is life-long and complete avoidance of gluten. Once gluten is removed from the diet the small bowel will repair and if a gluten-free diet is maintained, the small bowel will remain healthy and the absorption of nutrients will be normal.

Gluten-free foods include fresh fruit and vegetables such as potato, meat (except processed meats), poultry, fish and most dairy foods, rice, corn, sago, tapioca, buckwheat, soy and arrowroot.

Many carbohydrate rich, lower GI foods that help in managing diabetes are also sources of gluten

Your food intake must be well balanced and the amount and type of carbohydrate you choose to eat should help manage both your diabetes and coeliac disease.

Some of the carbohydrate foods promoted as being lower glycaemic index cannot be included in a gluten free diet. **You must avoid**:
- wheat- or rye-containing bread and cereals
- pasta
- barley
- rolled oats
- barley, wheat and oat brans

Good sources of carbohydrate that are lower in GI and are **suitable** for a gluten-free diet include:
- legumes (dried beans, peas, lentils)
- sweet potato
- sweet corn
- parsnip
- most fruit
- fresh rice noodles
- Mahatma™ long grain white, basmati, doongara rice
- milk and yoghurt
- millet
- buckwheat

- wild rice
- corn/maize starch
- quinoa

Gluten free, high carbohydrate, high GI foods include:
- potato
- tapioca/cassava
- arrowroot
- sago
- amaranth
- lupin
- sorghum

Fibre is often lacking in gluten free diets. Appropriate gluten free, good sources of fibre include:
- legumes (pulses)
- sweet potato
- sweet corn
- fruit
- millet
- buckwheat
- rice bran
- psyllium husks
- linseeds

These foods should be eaten regularly as individual foods or added to breads and cereals.

There are several food products available in supermarkets and specialist food shops that are suitable for people with diabetes and coeliac disease. These include breads and bread mixes, biscuits, cereals and pastas. Useful products include baked beans and corn tortillas but always check the label to make sure you choose gluten-free ones. Advice should be sought from a dietitian who can advise you on the suitability of these products and help you combine your dietary requirements with your food preferences.

Management is a team affair

In managing these combined conditions, regular consultations with your family doctor, specialists (usually endocrinologist and gastroenterologist or paediatrician), diabetes educator and dietitian are essential. Your insulin, diet and exercise must be well balanced to achieve good blood glucose management.

Hypoglycaemia must be treated quickly and immediately with carbohydrate

Poorly managed coeliac disease can lead to poorly managed diabetes and hyper glycaemia or hypoglycaemia. Hypoglycaemia must be treated quickly and immediately with carbohydrate. You should always carry some quickly absorbed, gluten-free form of carbohydrate with you to use in emergencies.

Pregnancy and diabetes

Diabetes should not stand in the way of a normal, healthy pregnancy. If you have diabetes, make sure it is well managed before you become pregnant. You will find both your nutritional needs and insulin dosage may change while you are pregnant. Get expert help from a dietitian, diabetes educator and diabetes specialist and have your diabetes reviewed frequently during your pregnancy so your baby gets the best possible start and you maintain your health throughout.

Long periods without food may increase the risk of ketosis

You may also need to change the timing of your carbohydrate intake at this time, to help with management of your diabetes. It is particularly important that you eat regular meals, especially breakfast and a bedtime snack. Long periods without food may increase your risk of ketosis, which can be harmful to you and to your baby.

A general recommendation during pregnancy is to use artificial sweeteners sparingly and to avoid products sweetened with saccharin and cyclamate. Diabetes Australia state that the following may be used in small amounts: Aspartame (Nutrasweet™, Equal™), Sucralose (Splenda™), Isomalt, Acesulphame K and Alitame (Aclame™). See page 67 for information on other artificial sweeteners.

Diabetes developed during pregnancy (gestational diabetes) may require insulin

Some women develop diabetes for the first time during pregnancy, usually between the twenty-sixth and twenty-eighth week. Hormones, produced by the pancreas, prevent the body's insulin from working properly and insulin injections are frequently necessary to ensure good blood glucose management. If diagnosed as having diabetes, you must take care of your diet throughout the remainder of your pregnancy to ensure that you and your baby are healthy.

Once the baby is born, the symptoms of diabetes may disappear, and reappear in later pregnancies. Approximately 50% of women who develop gestational diabetes develop Type 2 diabetes within twenty years and as time progresses diabetes is evident in 65% of these women.

You can help delay the onset of diabetes in later life by continuing a healthy eating plan, keeping a healthy weight and exercising regularly liafter the birth of your baby. This means you should act as if you still have diabetes.

Childhood and adolescence

Avoid making diabetes the focus of family life—it's just one aspect.

As children and adolescents develop, their dietary needs and insulin requirements will vary. It is important to have your child or adolescent's diet reviewed at least annually and their diabetes and general health monitored regularly

Food has important social implications for children and adolescents

As for all of us, food has important social implications for children and adolescents. While instilling in your child or teenager the enjoyment of a healthy eating plan, you may have to compromise at times. Food and eating should not become a battlefield, a focus of rebellion or a source of family tension. The entire family would benefit by eating in exactly the same way. Not only will the family benefit from the healthy diet, it will remove your child's sense of 'being different' or being deprived.

Teach your children the benefits of regular meals and a healthy way of eating. Encourage your child to see healthy eating as a positive aspect of life rather than as a negative aspect of having diabetes. Children should learn that diabetes does not mean being punished or deprived of food. Denying your child any sweet foods can lead to secret eating and binges. Don't make a fuss about fatty or sweet foods; remember that the occasional splurge will not cause any long-term harm.

Don't force your child to eat

It's easy to fall into the trap of replacing uneaten fruit, vegetables, breads and cereals with sugary foods because of a fear of hypoglycaemia. Children will soon learn to manipulate and may start refusing their meals, knowing you may offer them a sweet treat instead. Try offering healthy alternatives in this situation, such as fruit, milk or wholegrain bread. Do not create a habit of offering a range of alternative foods when they do not eat what you first offer. Children's appetites vary considerably from day to day and month to month. Don't force your child to eat; you don't always feel hungry and neither do they. Forcing a reluctant child to eat leads to resentment, rebellion and anxiety for everyone. You may find that, in the name of co-operation and family well-being, you have to sometimes make a temporary compromise on diabetes management for the sake of the long-term outcome.

Adolescence, with hormonal changes and growth spurts, brings its own special needs

Hormonal changes and growth spurts during adolescence may upset diabetes management even though your teenager is following the correct advice. It may be that their whole management routine needs a fresh appraisal. Adolescents need to realise how vital it is to seek medical help the moment they do not feel well. Failure to do this is a common cause of hospital admissions for poorly managed diabetes in this age group.

The teens are a time of exploration, testing and a desire for independence

The teens are a time of exploration, testing and a desire or need for independence. This applies to the issue of food just as much as it does to other realms of behaviour. If your teenager has a good knowledge of diabetes management, they will know how to be flexible in terms of mealtimes, foods eaten and the amount of insulin they need and when they need it. This may cause you considerable anxiety, but you must learn to encourage your child's sense of independence; allow them to learn by their own mistakes. For adolescents, the peer pressure to drink alcohol may be strong. Make sure your teenager understands how vital it is for them to have plenty of carbohydrate if they drink alcohol.

Teenagers should be encouraged to carry identification stating they have diabetes

Teenagers should be encouraged to carry identification stating they have diabetes, although some may rebel against this. It is often a time when it is most needed. The changes that may occur in diabetes management and the desire to experiment may affect diabetes management. Swings in blood glucose levels may result in behaviours that can be mistakenly interpreted as rebellious or lead to emergency hospital admissions. Close friends should be made aware that your teenager has Type 1 diabetes.

Children and adolescents like to snack

Children and adolescents like to snack, so prepare healthy and delicious snacks in advance to reduce the likelihood of them eating convenience and takeaway foods.

Children should take an active part in their diabetes management

With young children, it is important that they take an active part in their diabetes management, including blood glucose monitoring, insulin injections, food choices and planning meals. You will find that the more involved your child is, the less tension is likely to arise. By learning to monitor their own blood glucose level, your child will soon learn the effects of different foods. The better your child understands his or her diabetes, the more responsibility they will take for it and so they will cope better with their own changing needs as they grow older.

Children must learn to manage their diabetes when away from home

Make sure parents of friends and teachers at school know that your child has diabetes and that they know how to cope with hypoglycaemia and sickness. Diabetes is not a barrier to normal childhood activities such as parties, sport, staying at friends', trips or school camps and you should encourage your child to take part. Encourage your child to carry extra snacks, especially when they will be away from home for long periods such as sleeping out on weekends or going to after-school activities.

Let your child know that there are other children with diabetes. They are neither alone nor unique. Diabetes camps are an excellent way to reduce any sense of isolation. For details of these camps, get in touch with Diabetes Australia or the local children's hospital.

There are lots of ideas in this book for children and teenagers parties and school lunches

This book gives you lots of ideas for school lunches and for children and teenagers parties. In particular, see Special occasion meals pages 260–273, Lunches and light meals, pages 88–119 and Snacks pages 78–87.

For more lunch ideas visit:
- Go for Your Life at www.goforyourlife.vic.gov.au
- Better Heath Channel at www.betterhealthchannel.vic.gov.au

Diabetes and older people

To remain healthy as you grow older, it is important to eat well and remain as active as possible. A well-balanced eating plan helps prevent the changes associated with ageing such as loss of muscle, weakening of bones and decreasing energy levels.

Most people find their appetite decreases as they grow older, which may mean that smaller quantities of food are eaten. With diabetes, it is important that this food provides all the nutrition that you need and helps you maintain good blood glucose management. To do this it may become necessary to eat more of the foods that were limited when you were younger such as full-cream milks and regular cheeses.

A low-fat diet is often not suitable for older, underweight or frail people

Heart disease is a major cause of ill health in Australia and a low-fat diet is generally recommended. This is often not suitable for older, underweight or frail people as it may lead to excessive weight loss and limit the nutrients you eat. Unless you need to lose weight, it is wise to avoid a very low-fat diet while maintaining healthy choices and use poly- or mono- unsaturated margarines and oils when preparing foods.

If your appetite is limited, eat small amounts frequently

Make your meals interesting, enjoyable and well balanced by eating a variety of foods each day. If your appetite is limited choose small servings of foods and eat more frequently. It is usually best to have one main and two lighter meals daily with small nutritious snacks or drinks in between. Eat your main meal at the time of day when your appetite is best. For many people this is in the middle of the day.

Include your favourite dishes, add plenty of flavour to foods and serve a variety of colours to make your meals look attractive. Eat meals with family and friends whenever you can; social eating is fun.

Don't fill up on tea, bread and butter

It is often easy to have a cup of tea with bread and butter or biscuits, especially if you live alone. These may be filling but will not give you the nutrients you need. Include protein rich foods, vegetables and carbohydrate foods in each meal and use fruit and dairy foods in desserts. Eat 'treats' at the end of the meal if you wish.

Short-term and long-term illness (like cancer or depression) may decrease your appetite. If this is a concern for you, discuss your eating with your doctor or dietitian.

Decreased saliva production is part of the ageing process and a dry mouth often means chewing and swallowing becomes difficult. Make sure meats are tender and foods moist and soft. A little gravy or sauce will make swallowing easier. It is important to visit your dentist regularly. Missing teeth and poorly fitting dentures can make eating difficult.

Many prescription medications can effect appetite and taste of food

Ask your doctor about the medications prescribed for you. Some may decrease your appetite, cause nausea or change the way you taste your food. Others can cause constipation.

Eating plenty of high-fibre foods will help prevent constipation

Constipation can be a problem with many older people. Eating plenty of high-fibre foods such as fruits, vegetables, wholegrain breads and cereals, plus physical activity and drinking plenty of fluids will help you avoid constipation.

Your doctor may advise you to decrease the salt you add to meals

Salt adds to the taste of food and many older people enjoy salty foods like bacon, ham and cheese. Sometimes your doctor may advise you to cut down your salt intake for medical reasons.

Unless advised otherwise by your doctor, drink plenty of fluids

Drink at least six to eight cups of fluid every day. These can be water, tea, coffee, milk or fruit juice. Drink alcohol in moderation and always with food and remember that some medications will increase the effects of alcohol.

A good calcium intake, vitamin D and regular weight-bearing exercise will help maintain bones

To maintain strong bones, it is important to have plenty of calcium, vitamin D and regular weight-bearing exercise. Dairy foods provide the best sources of calcium. Vitamin D is made in your body when the skin is exposed to sunlight. It is a good idea to spend at least half an hour outdoors several times a week. You do not need direct sunlight; sitting in the shade or walking on a cloudy day is enough. Regular walking is a great way to help maintain healthy bones.

It is better to be a little overweight than underweight in your later years

If you are concerned that you are underweight or if you are unintentionally losing weight, seek help from a dietitian. They can make suggestions to help you.

Most local councils provide a home meal delivery service. These services can provide meals to suit individual needs, including diabetes and soft, pureed or cut up meals.

A good day's intake for older people is shown is the meal plan opposite. Vary the size of serves to suit your appetite. The carbohydrate-rich foods have been highlighted for easy identification.

Vegetarians with diabetes

A vegetarian eating-pattern needs to be well balanced, whether you have diabetes or not. It is important to plan your diet to ensure all nutrients are included in adequate amounts. The nutrients that may be lacking in a poorly planned vegetarian diet are protein, calcium, iron, zinc, cyanocobalamin (Vitamin B12) and riboflavin (B2).

It is easier to meet nutrient needs in a lacto-ovo diet than a vegan eating pattern

If you include dairy products and eggs in your vegetarian eating-plan (a lacto-ovo vegetarian diet) your nutrient needs can be easily met. If you choose not to eat any animal products (a vegan diet), it is best to consult a dietitian, who will help you plan an adequate eating pattern.

Breakfast

Fruit juice

Cereal—preferably wholegrain, like porridge made from rolled oats, Oatbix™, All bran™, wheatflakes, branflakes or muesli served with **milk**, **yoghurt** or **fruit**.

Toast—wholemeal or rye with margarine and a spread like Vegemite, peanut butter, marmalade, **jam** or **honey**.

Drink—water, tea, coffee, a **milk** drink

Morning tea

Fruit—fresh, cut up, or stewed

Snack such as a plain **biscuits**, a **muffin**, or a **scone** with margarine and jam

Drink—water, tea, coffee, a **milk** drink, **fruit juice**

Lunch/Dinner/Main meal

Cooked meat, chicken, fish or egg

Potato, **rice** or **pasta**

Vegetables, including **starchy** and non starchy

Dessert like **fruit**, **custard** or **baked dessert**

Drink—water, tea, coffee, a **milk** drink, **fruit juice**

Afternoon tea

Snack such as a **dry biscuit** with cheese, tomato, dip, a **scone** or **muffin**, **cake**—fruit, banana, carrot

Drink—water, tea, coffee, **milk** drink, **fruit juice**

Tea/Light meal

Soup—homemade, canned or packet

Sandwich—cheese, egg, meat, canned fish with side salad or a light dish—egg, baked beans on **toast**

Dessert—**fruit** and **custard**, **yoghurt**, **ice-cream**

Drink—water, tea, coffee, a **milk** drink, **fruit juice**

Supper

Drink—a **milk** drink, **fruit juice**, water, tea, coffee

Snack like a **biscuit** or **toast** with spread

It is fine to eat your main meal at either midday or in the evening, depending on what suits your lifestyle.

Sources of nutrients for vegetarian eating-patterns include:

- **Protein:** milk and milk products, eggs, pulses, nuts, seeds and cereal products. As the proteins from plant sources do not contain the complete set of amino acids the body requires, you should eat a variety of these products every day.
- **Calcium:** milk and milk products, sesame and sunflower seeds, tahine, almonds. Other plant foods contain small amounts of calcium
- **Iron and zinc:** pulses, wholegrain cereal products and green leafy vegetables and eggs
- **Riboflavin (B2):** milk and milk products, yeast extract (e.g. Vegemite™, Promite™, Marmite™), dried fruits, pulses, nuts and green leafy vegetables
- **Cyanocobalamin (Vitamin B12):** milk and milk products, eggs

Fortified soy milk is important for nutrients for people following a vegan eating-pattern

All soy milks are good sources of protein and many are fortified with calcium and some with riboflavin and cyanocobalamin (B12). It is worthwhile checking the label when buying soy milk. Calcium needs are hard to meet if a calcium fortified soy milk is not included regularly in the diet. A Vitamin B12 supplement is often recommended for people following a vegan lifestyle.

> **Read the labels when buying soy milk**
> Regular soy milks are poor sources of calcium, riboflavin (B2) and cyanocobalamin (B12) so buy products that are fortified with these nutrients.

Iron, particularly from vegetable sources, is not easily absorbed

The iron in plant foods is more difficult to absorb than iron from animal foods such as meat. Absorption is increased when foods with Vitamin C are eaten at the same meal. For instance, eat citrus fruits, pineapple, tomatoes or juice along with iron-rich foods such as cereal products, spinach or silverbeet. The tannin in tea interferes with the absorption of iron into your body, so don't finish your meal with a cup of tea. Fibre slows the absorption of many vitamins and minerals but this is counterbalanced by a well-balanced intake of foods.

Recommended daily food intake for lacto-ovo vegetarians

Milk and dairy products:

Three serves of dairy foods:

- 1 cup (250ml) milk = 40g hard cheese = 1 tub (200g) yoghurt
- low-fat cheeses, such as cottage and ricotta, are lower in calcium than full-cream cheeses
- all low-fat milks and regular milks provides good sources of calcium

Other protein-rich foods

Two serves of the following:

- eggs: 1 serve = 2 eggs
- pulses: 1 serve = ¾ cup (165g)
- nuts: 1 serve = 90g
- soy bean curd (tofu): 1 serve = 1 cup (220g)

Other foods

- fruit: at least 2–3 serves
- vegetables: at least 5 serves
- bread and cereals: a minimum of 4 serves or more, according to appetite
- fats: 1–2 tablespoons, including unsaturated oils and margarine

Exercise, sport and diabetes

Regular exercise is important for everyone who wants to achieve and maintain good health. In people with diabetes, it will improve the effectiveness of insulin and help in the management of blood pressure, blood fats and weight.

Always check with your doctor before starting a new activity program to make sure it is safe for you. For most, 30 minutes a day at least 5 times a week is recommended. This is not a call to become a super-athlete; brisk walking, swimming, gardening, bike riding, Tai Chi, yoga, weightlifting or aerobics are just some of the forms of exercise that are good.

Thirty minutes a day can be accumulative, it does not need to be achieved in one block, for example you may do 15 minutes of activity in the morning and another 15 minutes later in the day.

If you are not used to exercising, start slowly and stop if you feel any discomfort. To know whether your body is benefiting from exercise, check your pulse immediately afterwards; it should be faster than your usual resting level.

Regular exercise helps keep blood glucose levels within normal range

For people with diabetes, exercise helps keep blood glucose levels within normal range. People with Type 2 diabetes can improve the management of their diabetes and minimise their need for medication by exercising or playing sport regularly. If you have Type 1 diabetes, regular exercise is important, but requires more careful planning.

You will learn from experience how your body reacts to exercise and how best to balance your energy expenditure with the needs of your diabetes.

For the person without diabetes, the body is able to keep blood glucose levels constant during sport through the release of insulin and other hormones. When exercise begins, the body normally stops releasing insulin and produces hormones that stimulate the liver to release glucose into the blood. The insulin already present in the bloodstream allows the exercising muscles to take up the glucose, converting it to energy and keeping the blood glucose level constant.

As the exercise continues, the blood glucose level rises and the liver stops releasing glucose. The body then releases insulin again, so that more glucose can pass into the exercising muscle. This complex mechanism ensures that the blood glucose level normally remains constant.

In Type 1 diabetes, you cannot regulate the action of injected insulin

If you have Type 1 diabetes, you don't have the benefit of this natural regulation. Once you have taken your insulin injection, you cannot regulate its action. This means that you may have a wide variation in your blood glucose level during and after exercise. However, if you have enough insulin in your system and your blood glucose level is within the normal range at the start of exercise, then you can safely exercise.

If you don't have enough insulin available in your system when you begin exercising—in other words, your blood glucose level is high—your body can misread the situation and release more glucose into your bloodstream from the liver. Because you don't have enough insulin, the glucose can't pass into your muscle cells. As a result, your blood glucose level will rise excessively (hyperglycaemia). So check your glucose levels before you begin. **You shouldn't exercise if your blood glucose is above 15 mmol/L as your levels may rise even further**.

If, on the other hand, you have too much insulin in your blood and your blood glucose level is low, eat some carbohydrate before you begin to exercise and check your blood glucose level.

Hypoglycaemia while exercising

Hypoglycaemia is the most common concern for people on diabetes medication who exercise regularly. However, there are some simple steps you can take to help prevent this problem.

Become familiar with the effect exercise has on your blood glucose level

There are a few ways to become familiar with the effect exercise has on you:
- Check your blood glucose level before you exercise, especially if you are new to diabetes. If your level is low (below 6mmol/L), take a carbohydrate snack before you begin exercising. It is useful to take another test after the exercise, or during prolonged exercise. This way you will become familiar with the effect exercise has on your blood glucose level.

- If you are doing prolonged exercise you may need to take some carbohydrate food or drink during your activity.
- If you have been doing vigorous or prolonged exercise, your blood glucose level may continue to drop for up to 24 hours after you stop exercising, so you should eat some carbohydrate afterwards, too. You may also need to increase the carbohydrate in your next meal or snack.
- If you are exercising away from home, make sure you have some carbohydrate foods with you such as fruit, fruit juice, jelly beans or biscuits.
- You may also need to have a drink of water nearby to sip if you start to feel thirsty, and always protect yourself from the sun.
- Be aware of dehydration, but don't confuse this with hypoglycaemia as symptoms can be similar. If you exercise vigorously, especially in hot weather, keep drinking plenty of fluids before, during and after you exercise.
- When your exercise session is over, quench your thirst with a non-alcoholic drink. Alcohol may lower your blood glucose level further and also has a dehydrating effect.

Serious athletes with diabetes (and there are many) ensure that their diabetes is well managed before they begin training. Training is the time to fine-tune management. This will ensure peak performance during competition and support effective and rapid recovery.

Your food, medications and timing may need to be adapted to suit the type of sporting activity you do. Discuss your training and performance schedule with you doctor, dietitian and/or diabetes educator. They can work with you to manipulate the balance between food, insulin and activity. The only way to do this properly is to monitor your blood glucose level before, during and after you exercise and experiment until you are confident about the combination which suits your needs best.

Eating to suit your needs

Having regular meals spaced evenly over the day, instead of having only one or two big meals a day, will generally help you manage your blood glucose level better. Include carbohydrate with all meals and try to be relatively consistent with the amount of carbohydrate you eat. Include at least one low glycaemic index food per meal. How much food and carbohydrate food you eat will depend on your requirements. For example, a person doing a lot of physical activity will generally require more food and carbohydrate than someone who is relatively inactive.

Having diabetes does not mean you need to go hungry!

If you are restricting your food or carbohydrate intake to keep your blood glucose levels well managed and this is causing hunger or unintended weight loss, speak to your dietitian or diabetes educator about a healthy eating pattern to suit your needs. You may also need medical review.

Carbohydrate-rich foods have been highlighted in this simple meal plan

On the opposite page we have a simple meal plan which shows you how to put into practise the information we have given. The carbohydrate-rich foods have been highlighted for easy identification. The quantities of food will vary from person to person. Your age, activity level and your weight should guide you.

This menu is plain but shows how to distribute your carbohydrate evenly through the day.

Eating out

If you enjoy eating meals away from home you need to understand your diabetes and how to manage it when you eat out. If eating at a friend's house, you may have no control over the food served. Ask for more carbohydrate if you need to but don't worry if the food is not the same as you normally eat. Plan to return to your usual pattern at the next meal. On special occasions, a splurge won't cause any harm. If you eat out regularly however, then you will need to learn how to make suitable food choices.

Breakfast

- 1 serve wholegrain **cereal** with low-fat **milk**
- 1 serve **fruit**
- 1–2 slices wholegrain **toast** or rye **bread** with a scrape of margarine and a topping of your choice

Lunch

- 2 slices wholegrain or rye **bread** or **bread roll** with a scrape of margarine
- 1 thin slice of lean red meat or chicken (no skin) or tuna or salmon or egg or cheese
- plenty of salad vegetables
- 1–2 serves **fruit** and/or **yoghurt** or **custard**

Dinner

- 1 small serve lean red or white meat or fish
- 2 serves **starchy vegetables** and/or **pasta** or **rice**
- plenty of non-starchy vegetables
- 1–2 slices wholegrain or rye bread with a scrape of margarine
- 1 serve **fruit** and/or **yoghurt** or **custard**

Bedtime snack

- 1 serve wholegrain or heavy **fruit bread** or wholemeal **biscuit**, a scrape of margarine and/or
- 1 cup low-fat **milk** as drink

If on insulin injections, plan the timing of your injection to suit the meal

You may find the meal is served later than you are used to. If on insulin injections, you may postpone your injection until your meal is being served. Make sure you order enough carbohydrate with your meal or if there is likely to be more carbohydrate in the meal than you usually eat, consider increasing your insulin dose. If unsure about how to do this, discuss it with your doctor or diabetes educator.

Finding your way around the menu

Meals out don't have to be dull. Most restaurants will serve meals that fit into a healthy eating plan. The waiter can tell you what is in dishes if you are unsure. Don't be afraid to ask for meals to be prepared with minimal fat and for dressings and sauces to be served separately. If the restaurant foods seem high in kilojoules (calories), you may be wise to limit yourself to a starter and main course, or to a main course and dessert. The following ideas may get you started:

Soups

Thickened and 'creamed' soups will give you carbohydrate, but may be high in fats too. Ask the waiter to leave out the cream, or ask for a clear soup or a minestrone.

Entrees (starters)

Good choices are fresh oysters, vegetable parcels, skewered meats, seafood on rice, simple salads, asparagus spears or pasta with vegetable sauce. Avoid battered foods or foods served in rich sauces.

Main courses

Select small servings of lean chicken, fish, meat or seafood. An entree sized serve is often adequate. Avoid fried and battered foods and dishes loaded with cream, butter or cheese. To accompany your main course choose pasta, potato or rice to give you plenty of carbohydrate, and order vegetables or salads to add variety, flavour and colour and to help bulk up the meal if you are hungry.

Bread

If you want, ask for extra bread, but try to avoid high-fat garlic or herbed breads.

Desserts

These are often high in fat. If having something sweet to end a meal is important for you, ask for fruit, a simple fruit dessert, a sorbet, crème caramel or hot soufflé served without cream or rich sauces. You can also ask for a small serving or share a dessert with a friend.

Beverages

Limit your alcohol intake and don't be afraid to ask for a jug of iced water or soda water.

Different cuisines

There are many different cuisines to try:
- *Chinese*: short soup, combination of seafood or meat and vegetables or whole fish in ginger, steamed vegetables, steamed rice, plain noodles. Avoid fried rice, battered foods and sweet and sour dishes.
- *Greek*: dolmades, yoghurt or bean dips, grilled marinated meat, souvlaki, tabbouleh or green salad without dressing, plain pita bread.
- *Indian*: tandoori chicken or fish, raita, lean meat, fish, vegetable curry, chappatis, plain naan, steamed rice.

- *Italian*: minestrone or vegetable soup, pasta with a seafood or tomato sauce or a grilled fish or meat, green salad, crusty bread, fruit platter.
- *Japanese*: miso soup, sushi, nori or California rolls, meat/fish vegetable dishes. Avoid battered foods.
- *Mexican*: burritos, enchiladas or tostadas, less meat but more bean based dishes, green salad with salsa, refried beans, plain tortillas. Limit cheese, avoid sour cream.
- *Thai*: clear soup with noodles, steamed rolls, meat/fish vegetable or salads dishes.

Takeaway meals
These are often high in fat and salt. The following are better choices in terms of less fat:
- sandwiches, rolls or filled pita bread, ask for wholegrain or rye bread and no butter
- hamburger (plain meat and salad), avoid cheese and bacon
- jacket potatoes (without the sour cream)
- souvlaki
- barbecued or char-grilled chicken (no skin), salad and bread roll
- steamed dim sum
- noodles
- thin, crispy based pizza (order with less cheese, choose seafood or vegetarian or many of the wood fired, gourmet style)
- grilled fish, asked to be cooked in minimal oil, choose a small serve of thick chips or wedges.

Where possible, order fresh salad or fruit to balance the meal.

Occasional treats
Religious or feast days, birthdays and other family get-togethers are especially enjoyable and may include foods which are less suitable for good diabetes management. If you are the host, choose special recipes from this book for just such occasions. If you are a guest, have a little of the dishes you like, but balance this with vegetables, salad, bread and fruit.

A splurge now and then, on special occasions, does no harm; it's what you do for the rest of the time that counts. Return to your usual eating pattern at the next meal. Frequent splurging will contribute to weight gain and poorly managed diabetes.

This book gives you lots of ideas for those special parties and dinners. In particular, see Special occasion meals pages 260–273 and Lunches and light meals pages 88–119.

Some of your favourite recipes may seem unsuitable if you have diabetes, but before putting them away, see if you can alter them by using less fat and sugar, by increasing the fibre or adding low GI ingredients.

Add extra fruit, vegetables or legumes to recipes, for example:

- substitute half of the mince meat in a spaghetti bolognaise recipe with red kidney beans or chopped fresh vegetables
- double the amount of fruit in a fruit crumble

Use wholegrain flours or cereals where possible, for example:

- replace some of the white flour with wholegrain flour in muffins and fruit-based cakes. add a little more liquid if mixture seems too dry
- add a few tablespoons of barley or oat bran to bread, biscuit or muffin recipes

Use less saturated fat, for example:

- replace full-cream milk with skim or low-fat milk
- use margarine or oil instead of butter and reduce the quantity.

Where a recipe specifies that you cream the butter (margarine) and sugar, add the sugar to the dry ingredients and rub in the butter (margarine). Where you reduce butter and sugar in a recipe, it will not rise as high, and the texture will be a little denser. Try using a smaller baking tin.

If a favourite recipe can't be modified, use it for special occasions

Some recipes simply don't look and taste the same if modified. Put these on your list of occasional dishes and keep them as treats.

Travelling across time zones

When you are travelling short distances, try to have your meals at the normal times. When travelling by car, carry dry biscuits and fresh or dried fruit to eat if there are delays.

Overseas travel may mean a change in your normal eating pattern, particularly when you travel quickly across time zones. It is advisable to notify the airline in advance and request additional fresh fruit, breads, sandwiches and dry biscuits. If you are going to cross time zones, discuss your insulin and food requirements with your doctor, dietitian or diabetes educator before you leave on the trip. When travelling in different countries, you can always find suitable food even if it is limited in variety.

Shift work

Shift workers may need to vary timing of meals and medications

If you are a shift worker, the timing of your meals and medications may vary with the timing of your shifts. Because of the great variation in shifts and individual needs, it is difficult to give suggestions other than to strongly advise you to see a dietitian or diabetes educator for help. Basically you should aim to spread your meals and diabetes medication throughout your waking hours, just as you would on day shift—and treat the night as day. If you take your diabetes medication prior to going to bed, make sure that you have also eaten.

Eating to suit your needs

Making sense
of food labels

Food labels provide valuable information by stating the name of the product, the country of origin, the manufacturer or importer, a use-by or best-before date and a warning if the product contains any substance that may cause an allergic reaction, ingredients list and a nutrition panel.

The ingredients list

Food labelling laws in Australia state that all ingredients in a product must appear on the label, and in order of decreasing quantity by weight. This means the ingredient used in the greatest amount is listed first and that used in the smallest amount is listed last.

Fat, sugar, salt and fibre may be listed under different names. This means they may be difficult to recognise. Here are various ingredients listed under their food group.

Fat: Animal fat, beef fat, beef tallow, butter fat, cocoa fat, coconut cream, coconut oil, copha, corn oil, cottonseed oil, hydrogenated oil, lard, lecithin, margarine, oil, palm oil, shortening, soya bean oil, vegetable fat, vegetable oil.

Sugar: Apple concentrate, brown sugar, concentrated fruit juice, corn syrup, dextrose, disaccharides, fructose, glucose, glucose syrup, golden syrup, grape concentrate, honey, invert sugar, lactose, malt, malt extract, maltose, mannitol, modified carbohydrate, molasses, pear concentrate, raw sugar, sorbitol, sucrose, treacle, xylitol.

Salt: Celery salt, cooking salt, herb salt, lemon salt, lite salt, monosodium glutamate (MSG) or flavour enhancer 621, onion salt, rock salt, sea salt, sodium bicarbonate, sodium chloride, sodium nitrate, soy sauce, table salt, tenderizer, vegetable salt.

Fibre: Barley bran, bran, oat bran, psyllium husks, rice bran, rolled oats, wheat bran, wheatgerm, wheatmeal, wholegrain, wholemeal, wholewheat.

The nutrition panel

It is not just the order of the ingredients that is important when assessing the nutrient value of a food product but the amount of each ingredient. For instance, the second and third ingredient listed may help make up the bulk of the product, along with the first ingredient, or they may be there only in small amounts. It is therefore important to look for a nutrition information panel on the label of most product's.

The nutrition information panel shows the nutrient composition. This information allows you to make product comparisons. Information can include energy (kilojoule/calorie), protein, fat (and often types of fats), carbohydrate (often total and sugars), minerals, vitamins and fibre content. Amounts are given 'per recommended serving' and 'per 100g' or 'per 100ml'. The 'per 100g' is the most useful for comparing foods which are of similar type. Note that grams 'per 100g' are the same as percentage. For instance 3g fat per 100g of product means that the product is 3% fat.

Make healthy choices when buying foods

Make healthy food choices by checking the fat, sugar, fibre and salt contents of products. Use the chart below to compare products and, with the exception of fibre, consider these figures maximum amounts when making your choice. Make sure the food is palatable but don't be fooled into choosing a food low in one nutrient if it is high in another. For instance, you may find biscuits which are low fat but high in salt. A better choice would be biscuits which are low in both fat and salt.

Label example—Weet-Bix™

NUTRITION INFORMATION		PER SERVE 30g	PER 100g
Serving per package 24	Energy	447 kJ	1490 kJ
Serving size 30 g	Protein	3.7g	12.4g
	Fat - Total	0.4g	1.4g
	- Saturated	0.1g	0.3g
	Carbohydrates - Total	20.1g	67g
	- Sugars	1.0g	3.3g
	Dietary Fibre	3.3g	11.0g
	Sodium	87mg	290mg

INGREDIENTS: Wholegrain wheat, raw sugar, salt, barley malt extract, minerals, vitamins

In this product, sugar appears high on the list of ingredients, but on checking the nutrition information you can see that the amount of sugar per serve is quite low.

Weet-Bix™ has a medium–high GI, is high in fibre and low in fat.

Healthy choices when buying foods

Food product	Fat (g/100g)	Sugar (g/100g)	Fibre (g/100g)	Salt mg/100g
Dry biscuits	<5		>5	<350
Sweet biscuits	<5	<10		<250
Bread	<5		>5	<450
Breakfast cereals	<5	<15	At least 5, ideal >10	<400
Milk and yoghurt	<2	Milk <10 Yoghurt <15		<50
Cheese	<15, ideal <10			<600
Dairy desserts	<3	<15		
Meat	<10			
Margarine	<20 saturated fat, <1 trans fat, ideal nil			<400
Mayonnaise	<10			<750

(Adapted from Heart Foundation information)

Packaging claims

Claims that appear on the label of a package can often mislead. The following highlight some common claims, some have no legal definition but some do:

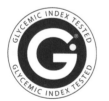

The GI Symbol

This useful symbol has been used on many packaged food products since 2002. It indicates the GI rating of the food. The foods which show the symbol have had their GI tested at an accredited laboratory. They meet strict guidelines to ensure they are not too high in kilojoules, saturated fat or sodium and where appropriate, they are a source of dietary fibre and calcium. Testing for GI is an expensive process and not all manufacturers can afford to have foods tested. With time, this symbol should appear on many more foods as their GI rating is tested.

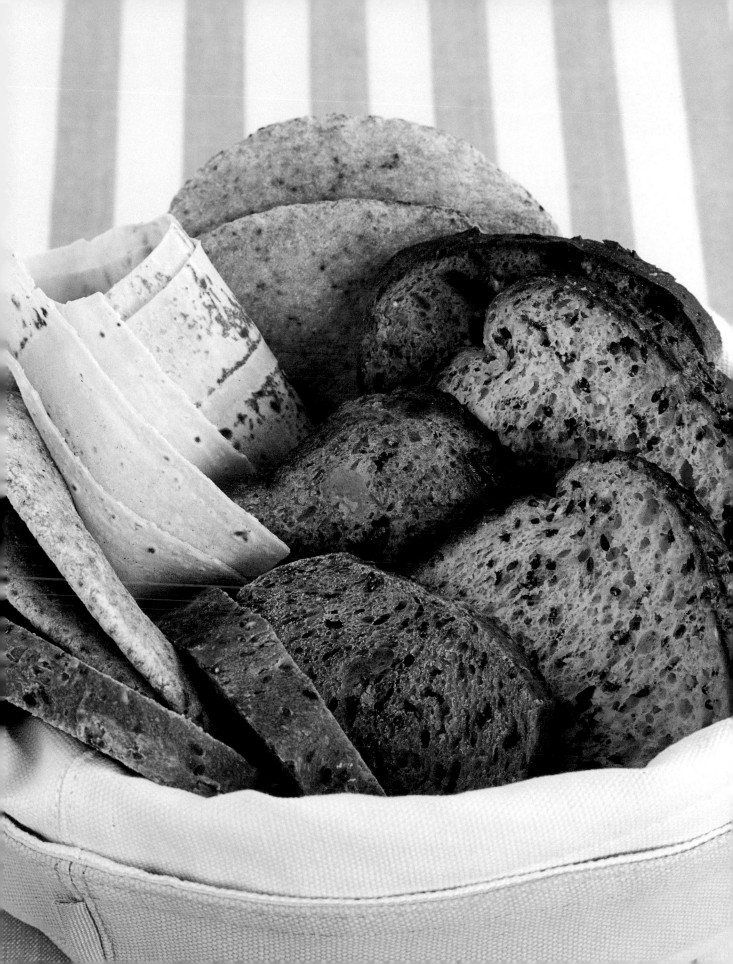

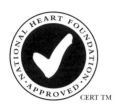

CERT TM

The Heart Foundation Tick

Foods with the Heart Foundation Tick have passed rigorous independent assessment in Australia. Random audits are carried out to ensure strict nutrition standards are maintained for things like saturated fat, trans fat, sodium, kilojoules (calories) and fibre. With more than 1200 foods in supermarkets, there's bound to be a healthier 'Tick' alternative to the foods you and your family eat every day. When you're looking for quick lunches and dinners away from home, look for Heart Foundation Tick approved meals that meet nutrition and promotion requirements and strict standards for food safety and preparation. Despite the cost to companies, the numbers of foods being assessed are increasing as the benefits of the Tick are recognised.

Light or lite

Can refer to colour, salt, fat, energy (kilojoules) or flavour, e.g. light olive oil is light in flavour not in total fat content.

Percentage fat-free

Not necessarily low in fat, e.g., an 80% fat-free cheese still means it has a 20% fat.

Percentage reduced fat or reduced fat

Does not mean the product is low in fat, e.g., a cheese which is reduced in fat by 30% may mean it has been reduced from 30% to 20% fat content.

No cholesterol, cholesterol-free, low cholesterol

Refers only to cholesterol content. These products may still be high in fat. All foods that originate from plants and their oils are free of cholesterol.

Sugar-free or no added sugar

Must not contain added common sugar (sucrose or cane sugar) but may be high in naturally occurring sugars such as fructose, lactose, grape juice, apple concentrate and pear juice. The energy (kilojoule) value of these products can be as high as regular sugar-sweetened products.

Low-joule

Must be much lower in kilojoules (calories) or energy value than their regular equivalent. These products may be of use to people who have diabetes and/or are overweight. Included are low-joule (calorie) jelly, soft drink and cordials and no-oil dressings.

Diabetic or carbohydrate modified

These products are targeted at people with diabetes. Some diabetic (carbohydrate modified) chocolate, ice-cream and biscuits are high in fat. Other products include jams, chutneys, pickles and sauces which are low in fat. Generally, you will find that these specialised products are more expensive and do not taste as good as the regular variety. It is often best to use the regular products sparingly.

All Natural

Can mean anything from using honey as a sweetener to organically grown or free of synthetic additives.

Artificial and alternative sweeteners

Some artificial or intense sweeteners have negligible kilojoules. These include: Aspartame (Equal™ or Nutrasweet™), Cyclamate, Saccharin and Sucralose (Splenda™), Acesulphame K and Aliame (Aclame™).

Other types of artificial and alternative sweeteners contain a similar amount of kilojoules to sugar (sucrose), including sorbitol, fructose and lactose. Mannitol contains half the amount of kilojoules than sugar.

Artificial sweeteners that contain negligible kilojoules can be used to lower kilojoule intake, for example an artificially sweetened can of soft drink contains very few kilojoules (375ml diet cola provides approximately 6 kilojoules/1 calorie) compared to a can of regular soft drink (375ml cola provides approximately 655 kilojoules/157 calories). Overall, however, a healthy diet is one that includes minimal processed foods and thus the role for artificial sweeteners is limited.

Artificial sweeteners can be advantageous in chewing gums because they do not contribute to tooth decay in the way that sugar does. Artificially sweetened soft drinks promote tooth decay in a similar way to regular soft drinks due to the high acid levels.

Recipes

Most of the recipes in this book are simple and quick to prepare and we have generally tried to avoid using ingredients that can be difficult to find.

GI value of recipes

We have used low GI ingredients where practical in the recipes and have provided advice before each section to help show you how to incorporate lower GI foods into your meals.

The glycemic index or GI value of a recipe can only be obtained accurately by testing the prepared meal in a laboratory. This is because the GI of food changes when combined with other ingredients or food items. For instance the addition of an acid food or the presence of fat decreases the GI of a dish. See page 22 for further information about GI.

We have, however, also rated the GI value of our recipes as low, medium or high using only the ingredients containing carbohydrate with known GI values. Where the carbohydrate content of a recipe is negligible i.e. equal to or less than 5 grams per serve we have not given the recipe a GI rating.

Nutrient value of recipes

The kilojoule (calories), carbohydrate, protein, total fat, saturated fat, sodium and fibre content are given for each recipe. Recipes have been analysed using FoodWorks (Xyris software).

Where a choice of ingredients is given in a recipe, the first one listed is the one we use in our analysis of nutritional value.

Salt

It may be important for you to decrease your salt intake especially if you have high blood pressure and/or if you have been advised to do so by your doctor. We recommend you use salt sparingly and when using commercial products to buy those with no added or reduced salt. We have done this for the analysis of all our recipes.

Fats

We use a number of ways to reduce the fat, and especially saturated fat, content of our recipes:

Oil: we have kept the oil to a minimum by using spray oil or where necessary a maximum of 1 tablespoon of oil in recipes that serve four.

Margarine: we frequently use margarine in our recipes but do not specify the type. It is recommended that poly- or mono-unsaturated, low salt margarine is used.

Milk: we use skim or low-fat milk (one to two per cent fat).

Yoghurt: we substitute low-fat natural yoghurt for full-cream yoghurt except where the result is greatly improved by using full-cream yoghurt.

Cheeses: we use low-fat cheeses:

- skim milk variety cottage cheese
- low-fat or smooth ricotta cheese
- low-fat tasty or block cheese (less than 18% fat)
- 80% fat reduced cream cheese
- a mixture of low-fat ricotta and low-fat cream cheese.

To enhance the flavour of some recipes, we include a small amount of higher fat tasty cheeses, such as parmesan. Here, we use the principle that a small amount goes a long way.

Coconut milk: we use low-fat evaporated canned milk with added coconut essence or low-fat coconut flavoured evaporated milk (available in supermarkets)

Sugar and other sweeteners

We use a variety of sweetening agents in our recipes, including sugar in small amounts, as this is unlikely to cause a significant rise in the blood glucose level. Some recipes, especially baked products, rely on sugar to produce good results.

You will also see that we use natural sweetening agents other than sucrose (table sugar), such as fruit juice and dried fruits. A range of artificial sweeteners can be used occasionally. Some of these are suitable for baking and cooking, some are not, so check the product label.

Measuring foods

Ingredients in this book are given in measuring spoons or cups or in both grams (g) and ounces (oz). Size is given in centimetres and inches.

If you want things to turn out well, we advise you to measure ingredients carefully.

You will need a set of standard Australian measuring cups (¼, ⅓, ½ and 1 cup) and a standard set of measuring spoons (¼, ½, and 1 teaspoon [5ml], and 1 tablespoon [20ml]). These are available at supermarkets and kitchenware suppliers.

We have used cup and spoon measures rather than weights to simplify reading of recipes and to help make preparation easier. Should you want to weigh ingredients, see list at back of this book for weight conversions.

Different countries use different standard measures

The standards for Australian measure in millilitres (ml):

1 teaspoon = 5ml; 1 tablespoon = 20ml; 1 cup = 250ml. All spoon and cup measurements are level.

In New Zealand, Canada, United States of America and the United Kingdom:

1 teaspoon = 5ml or 0.17 fluid ounce; 1 tablespoon = 15ml or 0.5 fluid ounce

In some countries, such as the United States of America:

1 cup measure = 240ml or 8 fluid ounces. This difference is only small and will not change the results of our recipes.

Oven temperatures

The accuracy of oven thermometers can vary. You learn to adjust the temperature given in recipes to suit your oven.

We have given oven temperatures in degrees Celsius (°C). If you use a fan forced oven, reduce the temperature by about 20 degrees. If you use degrees Farenheit (°F), double the temperature given or use the conversion chart below.

Equivalent oven temperatures:

	°C	°F	Gas mark
slow	150	300	2
moderate	180	350	4
moderately hot	190	375	4½
hot	200	400	5
very hot	230	450	6

Alternative names

Some of the foods and utensils in this book are called by different names. These are outlined in the table opposite.

Name	Alternative name	Name	Alternative name
Vegetable, pulse, fruits		**Other food items**	
bean shoots	bean sprouts	bicarbonate of soda	baking soda
beans, green	beans, French	biscuits, sweet	cookies
beetroot	round beets/red beets	biscuits, dry	crackers
capsicum	bell pepper, pepper	bisc, shredded wheatmeal	Graham crackers, Digestive
chickpeas	garbanzos, channa	scones	biscuits
chillies	chilli pepper	chocolate, cooking	chocolate, baking
canola oil	rapeseed oil	cocoa	cocoa powder
coconut, desiccated	shredded coconut	cream, single,	cream, half and half,
coriander	cilantro	essence	
eggplant	aubergine	(vanilla essence)	extract (vanilla extract)
kiwi fruit	Chinese gooseberry	flour, corn	cornstarch
marrow	summer squash	flour, plain	flour, all-purpose
onion, Spanish	onion, purple/red, Bermuda	flour, self raising	flour, self-rising
onion, spring	scallions, shallots	flour, whole meal	flour, whole wheat
onions, small,		jam	jelly, conserve, preserve
shallots	scallions, green onions	jelly	Jello
passionfruit	granadilla	milk, low fat	milk, semi-skimmed
paw paw	papaya	milk, skim	milk, skimmed
pine nut	pignoli	mixed spice	pudding spice
pumpkin	canned pumpkin	pikelets	griddle cakes
rock melon/		stock cubes	bullion cubes
canteloup	cantaloupe, rock melon	sugar, caster	sugar, fine granulated
snow peas	mange tout	sugar, icing	sugar, confectioners
spinach,		syrup, glucose	liquid glucose,
silverbeet	Swiss chard, seakale		corn syrup
sultanas	golden raisins	syrup, golden	syrup, corn
sweet potato		treacle	molasses
(orange)	kumara	Rice Bubbles	Rice Crispies
tomato sauce	ketchup or catsup		
zest, lemon, etc	zest or rind, lemon, etc		
zucchini	courgettes		
Meat, seafood, nut, seed		**Utensils & Equipment**	
banger/sausages	link sausage	baking tray	cookie sheet, oven slide
fish sauce	nam pla, nuoc nam	cake cooler	wire rack
fillet steak	eye fillet, beef tenderloin	cake tin	baking pan
ham	jambon	ring tin	tube pan
hazelnut	filbert	Swiss roll tin	jelly roll pan
minced beef/meat	ground beef/meat	Lamington tin	13" x 9" x 2" pan
peanut butter	peanut paste	patty cups	paper cupcake holders
pepitas	pumpkin seeds	tea towel	dish towel
prawn	shrimp	griller	
prawn, king	shrimp, jumbo	(separate from oven)	broiler (inside oven)
skirt steak	flank steak		
tahini	sesame seed paste	Serve	Serving

Breakfasts

Start your day with plenty of carbohydrate and fibre

Fuelling up at breakfast time is an important way to start the day and breakfast is an ideal time to eat some low GI, fibre-rich foods. Breakfast can be a quick meal or a more leisurely one. It does not need to be complicated to satisfy.

It can be as simple as a bowl of cereal and a serve of fruit; omelettes, with fillings such as low-fat cheese and herbs; tomato combined with lean ham and onion, or a mushroom sauce; or try fruit filled pancakes topped with yoghurt. (Pancake recipes can be found on page 148.) If you prefer a quickly prepared cooked meal, try toast made with rye or wheat wholegrain, soy and linseed, oats and barley, genuine sour dough breads, or bread displaying the GI symbol topped or served with:

- baked beans with freshly chopped mushrooms or capsicum
- tomatoes, asparagus, mushrooms or sweetcorn
- poached, scrambled or boiled eggs.

Fruit provides carbohydrate, fibre, vitamins and minerals

Fruit cleanses the palate and provides carbohydrate, fibre, vitamins and minerals. Most fruit is low in GI (see pages 23 and 279–280). Eat it fresh, stewed or canned in natural juice. Combine fruits, top them with low-fat yoghurt, cottage or low-fat ricotta cheese, add them to porridge or cereal, or eat them on their own.

Breakfast cereals are high in carbohydrate and can be a good source of fibre and low in GI

Breakfast cereal can be homemade or you can choose from commercial products available (see page 276). Porridge makes a terrific start to the day and can be cooked with sultanas, diced raw apple or pear, cinnamon or nuts.

Make your own breakfast blend using oats, all-bran, wheatgerm, bran (all sorts—rice, corn, oat, barley or wheat), dried fruits of every kind, unsalted raw nuts, seeds (pumpkin, sesame, linseed and sunflower), millet, buckwheat, puffed rice, wheat or corn and wheatflakes. Serve with hot or cold skim or low-fat milk, yoghurt and fruit.

Fruit crunch muesli

Makes 16 cups (32 serves)
1 serve = ½ cup
**This is quick to make,
about 10–15 minutes**

1kg (2lb) raw rolled oats

½ cup moist flaked coconut

1 cup sultanas

1 cup chopped dried apricots

2 cups barley bran (or oat bran)

1 cup coarsely chopped brazil nuts

¼ cup sunflower seeds or pepitas

Method

1. Mix all ingredients well with a large spoon or your fingers.
2. Allow ⅓ cup per serve. Store in an airtight container.

Nutrition data per serve:
912 kJ (218 cal), carbohydrate 29g, protein 6g, fat 8g,
saturated fat 2g, fibre 5g, sodium 9mg
GI rating: low

Bircher muesli

Serves 6
**Preparation time: 20 minutes
+ overnight soaking of oats**

2 cups rolled oats

1½ cups orange juice

1 punnet fresh blueberries OR
300g (10½oz) frozen blueberries

1 green apple, grated

1 orange, peeled, segmented,
and the segments cut in half

1 cup low-fat natural
or fruit yoghurt

¼ cup chopped pecans

Tip: use regular rolled oats and
not 'quick' oats as
they are lower GI

Method

1. Place oats and juice in a bowl, mix well together
2. Cover with a lid or plastic wrap and chill overnight in
   refrigerator.
3. Before serving, add the grated apple, the orange, the
   berries, the pecans and the yoghurt and mix together.
4. Spoon into bowls

Variations

• You can replace the yoghurt with milk if you prefer
• The blueberries can be replaced with banana, other berries,
  dried fruit like apricots, pear or peaches, fresh pears, stone
  fruit in season
• Try other nuts—hazels, almonds
• Add spices like cinnamon, mixed spice, or ground cloves

Nutrition data per serve:
1043 kJ (248 cal), carbohydrate 38g, protein 6g, fat 7g, saturated
fat 0.7g, fibre 5g, sodium 20mg
GI rating: low

Fruit smoothie

This is a quick and easy way to start the day for people 'on the run' or with a small appetite—it is packed with nutrition and long lasting energy. So if you are short of time or find it hard to always eat breakfast, blending milk and fruit makes a nourishing replacement meal which provides plenty of carbohydrate and can be low GI.

Serves 2
Preparation time: 5 minutes

1½ cups skim or low-fat milk

½ cup low-fat natural yoghurt

2 bananas
or 1 cup fresh strawberries

1 egg (optional)

1–2 teaspoons sugar
OR artificial sweetener

Ground allspice, cinnamon
or nutmeg, for garnish

1 tablespoon psyllium

Method

1. Place all ingredients in a blender or food processor and mix well.
2. Serve at once, topped with a sprinkling of spice.

Variations:

- 1 ripe mango, peeled and flesh chopped
- 1 cup frozen or fresh berries—raspberries, mixed berries
- ½ cup passionfruit pulp
- 2–3 ripe kiwi fruit, peeled
- 2–3 fresh peaches or nectarines, peeled
- ½ cup canned fruit in natural juice

Nutrition data per serve:
1026 kJ (245 cal), carbohydrate 38g, protein 16g, fat 3g, saturated fat 1.0g, fibre 5g, sodium 167mg
GI rating: low

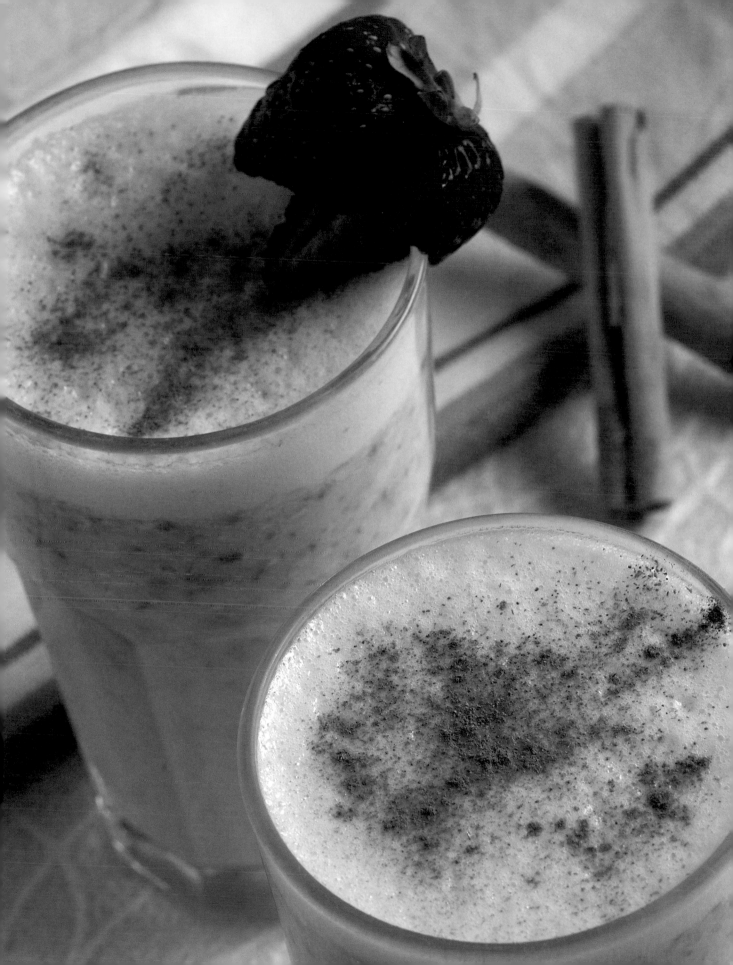

Apple and sultana pancakes

Serves 4
(2 pancakes per serve)
Preparation/cooking time:
10 minutes + preparation time
for pancakes

4 apples, peeled, cored and sliced

2 cloves

2 tablespoons sultanas

8 thick pancakes (see page 76),
warmed

4 rounded tablespoons
low-fat yoghurt

Method

1. Poach apples gently in a little water with cloves and sultanas for approximately 5 minutes until soft. Alternatively, microwave, covered, on high for 5–8 minutes.

2. Remove cloves and divide apple mixture evenly between pancakes.

3. Spoon warm mixture over the pancakes and top with a spoonful of low-fat fruit yoghurt.

Nutrition data per serve:
1727 kJ (413 cal), carbohydrate 70g, protein 12g, fat 8g, saturated fat 1.5g, fibre 7g, sodium 278mg
GI rating: low

Muffins make a change for breakfast and are good for those who take breakfast on the run or for those who like to relax with a coffee and the paper. See recipes pages 80–82.

French toast

This is an old-time favourite for children and adults alike. It is easy to prepare and children love helping to make it. Choose low GI bread and for a special breakfast with the children, cut bread into shapes with biscuit cutters.

Serves 4
Preparation/cooking time:
15 minutes

4 eggs

½ cup low-fat milk

Salt to taste (optional)

8 slices wholegrain or low GI white bread

2 teaspoons margarine

Optional for serving:
tomato relish, tomato sauce or
4 teaspoons caster or icing sugar

Method

1. Beat eggs with milk and a little salt in a large mixing bowl.
2. Cut slices of bread into halves (or with a biscuit cutter for children).
3. Heat a non-stick pan with a little of the margarine.
4. Dip the bread into the egg mixture, allowing the bread to absorb the mixture but not become too soggy, as it will fall apart.
5. Lightly brown on one side, turn and lightly brown on the other side. Repeat using the remaining margarine until all the bread is cooked.
6. Serve with tomato relish, a little tomato sauce or a fine sprinkling of caster or icing sugar.

Nutrition data per serve:
961 kJ (229 cal), carbohydrate 22g, protein 13g, fat 9g, saturated fat 2.2g, fibre 4g, sodium 335mg
GI rating: low

Snacks

Eating regularly and including snacks between meals can help even out blood glucose levels and satisfy appetite, but remember, snacking can contribute unnecessary kilojoules (calories) which, in turn, can lead to weight gain.

A dietitian or diabetes educator can advise you on the need for snacks in your eating plan.

If buying pre-made snacks, choose ones that are low GI or look for the GI symbol on products. The snack suggestions we give you are nourishing and use low GI ingredients.

Fruit

Any fruit is great as a snack, but the lower GI ones (see page 23 and 279–280) are ideal. If you like the higher GI fruits, then combine with lower GI varieties—fruit salad is a good example of this 'mix and match' approach. Grab a piece of fruit, make a fruit platter and serve with some low-fat natural or fruit yoghurt, enjoy a bowl of chopped fresh fruit or canned fruit in natural juice with yoghurt or low-fat custard. Dried fruit, especially dried apple, pears, sultanas, apricots and cranberries makes a good snack either eaten alone, or combined with some fresh fruit or nuts and/or seeds such as almonds, pecans, walnuts, pistachios, pepitas and sunflower seeds.

A milk drink

Try a smoothie see page 74, or simply mix milk with coffee or Milo™. Milk drinks are low GI and boost your calcium intake. In summer, an iced coffee made with low-fat milk and a scoop of low-fat ice-cream is simply delicious.

Dry biscuits

Add low-fat cheese and tomato, a scrape of peanut butter, some salsa (there are plenty of tasty low-fat tomato-based versions in the supermarket), or try our dip ideas on pages 250–254).

Bread or toast

If you are really hungry, a sandwich or a bowl of lower GI cereal with low-fat milk or yoghurt is hard to beat!

Cereal

Choose a GI cereal with low-fat milk or yoghurt.

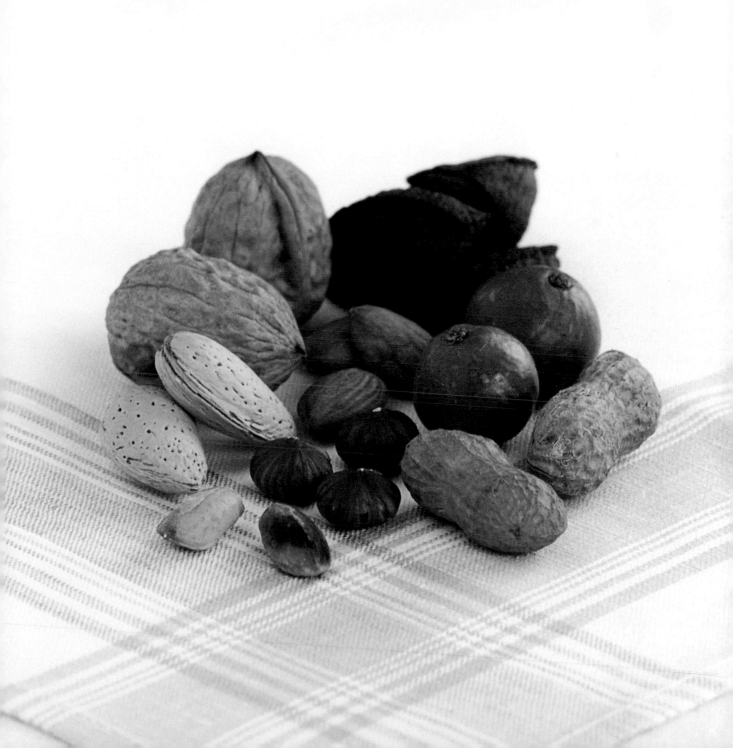

Muffins

Muffins can make a satisfying snack but can be very high in fat and/or added sugar, so we have given you a basic recipe with variations that are lower in fat and sugar but still delicious. Most muffins don't keep well, but you can freeze them to re-heat later in the oven or microwave.

By tradition, many baked products, especially pastries, cakes and biscuits, are high in fat, sugar and additives, and low in fibre and other nutrients. These days, however, the trend is often towards healthier foods and some good, lower GI breads, cakes, muffins and biscuits are now available commercially.

Basic savoury muffins

**Makes 12 muffins
(1 muffin per serve)
Preparation/cooking time:
30 minutes**

1¾ cups self-raising flour

½ teaspoon baking powder

2 tablespoons oat bran

1 cup low-fat milk

3 tablespoons margarine

1 egg, lightly beaten

Pepper and salt to taste
(optional)

Method

1. Preheat oven to 200°C (400°F).
2. Add the oat bran to the milk and allow to soak for 10–15 minutes while you continue with the recipe.
3. Sift the flour and baking powder into a large mixing bowl.
4. Heat the margarine until just melted, leave to cool a few minutes.
5. Grease the muffin tins—a light spray with oil in the base should be enough.
6. Add the beaten egg to the milk mixture and stir in well, then add the warm margarine and stir again.
7. Fold the flavourings into the flour, then pour the milk mixture into the bowl, fold gently and minimally with a metal spoon (it doesn't matter if the mixture looks lumpy!).
8. Then spoon into the muffin tins and put in the oven.
9. Muffins take 10–15 minutes to cook, but to check, if you touch the centre of one it should be lightly browned and firm to the touch.

Nutrition data per muffin:
515 kJ (123 cal), carbohydrate 17g, protein 4g, fat 4g, saturated fat 0.8g, fibre 1g, sodium 247mg
GI rating: low–med

Muffin variations

Herby Corn: 1 cup corn kernels, 1 teaspoon dried mixed herbs, 1 tablespoon chopped chives
2 tablespoons chopped parsley
Reduce flour to 1¼ cups, leave out the oat bran and increase baking powder to ¾ teaspoon
Add: ½ cup polenta (fine cornmeal)

Nutrition data per muffin:
554 kJ (132 cal), carbohydrate 18g, protein 4g, fat 5g, saturated fat 0.8g, fibre 1g, sodium 248mg
GI rating: med

Ham and cheese: 4 tablespoons freshly grated parmesan cheese, ¼ teaspoon paprika, ¼ teaspoon nutmeg, 2 tablespoons chopped parsley
Reduce margarine to 2 tablespoons
Add: 2 slices very lean ham, chopped finely

Nutrition data per muffin:
535 kJ (128 cal), carbohydrate 17g, protein 5g, fat 4g, saturated fat 1.0g, fibre 1g, sodium 322mg
GI rating: low–med

Sweet potato and spring onion: 4 spring onions, chopped finely, 1 tablespoon chopped parsley, ¼ cup grated low-fat tasty or block cheese
Reduce margarine to 2 tablespoons
Add: 1 cup cooked sweet potato, cut into small chunks

Nutrition data per muffin:
574 kJ (131 cal), carbohydrate 20g, protein 5g, fat 4g, saturated fat 1.0g, fibre 2g, sodium 253mg
GI rating: low–med

Basic sweet muffins

Makes 12 average-size muffins (1 muffin per serve) Preparation/cooking time: 30 minutes

1¾ cups self raising flour

½ teaspoon baking powder

2 tablespoons oat bran

1 cup low-fat milk

3 tablespoons raw sugar

3 tablespoons margarine

1 egg, lightly beaten

½ teaspoon vanilla essence

Nutrition data per muffin:
608 kJ (146 cal), carbohydrate 22g, protein 4g, fat 4g, saturated fat 0.8g, fibre 2g, sodium 249mg
GI rating: med

Method

1. Preheat oven to 200°C (400°F).
2. Add oat bran, vanilla and the sugar to the milk and allow to soak for 10–15 minutes while you continue with the recipe.
3. Sift flour, baking powder, plus any spices (see variations), into a mixing bowl.
4. Gently heat the margarine until melted, allow to cool a few minutes.
5. Grease the muffin tins—a light spray with spray oil in the base of the tins should be enough.
6. Add the beaten egg to the milk mixture and stir in well, then add the warm margarine and stir again.
7. Add the flavours to the flour, tossing lightly to dust the ingredients with flour, then pour the milk mixture into the bowl, fold lightly and minimally with a metal spoon (it doesn't matter if the mixture looks lumpy!), then spoon into muffin tins and put in the oven. Muffins take 10–15 minutes, but to check, touch the centre of one—it should be a little springy and lightly browned.

Variations:

Blueberry: 1 cup fresh or frozen blueberries + 1 teaspoon cinnamon

Nutrition data per muffin:
615 kJ (147 cal), carbohydrate 23g, protein 4g, fat 4g, saturated fat 0.8g, fibre 1g, sodium 249mg
GI rating: med

Apricot pecan: ¾ cup chopped dried apricots + ½ cup chopped pecans + ½ teaspoon mixed spice

Nutrition data per muffin:
819 kJ (196 cal), carbohydrate 25g, protein 5g, fat 8g, saturated fat 1.0g, fibre 2g, sodium 252mg
GI rating: low

Apple sultana: ½ cup sultanas + 1 large apple, peeled and grated + 1 teaspoon mixed spice

Nutrition data per muffin:
716 kJ (171 cal), carbohydrate 28g, protein 4g, fat 4g, saturated fat 0.8g, fibre 2g, sodium 252mg
GI rating: low

Raspberry: 1 cup fresh or frozen raspberries + 1 teaspoon grated lemon rind.

Nutrition data per muffin:
608 kJ (146 cal), carbohydrate 22g, protein 4g, fat 4g, saturated fat 0.8g, fibre 2g, sodium 249mg
GI rating: med

Apple scones

Makes 15 scones
(1 scone per serve)
Preparation/cooking time:
20 minutes

1 cup white flour

1 cup wholemeal flour

2 tablespoons sugar

½ teaspoon bi-carb soda

2 teaspoons baking powder

1 teaspoon mixed spice

3 tablespoons margarine

2 medium apples, peeled and cored—1 grated and 1 diced

½ cup low-fat or skim milk

½ teaspoon ground cinnamon

Method

1. Preheat oven to 220°C (425°F) and spray a baking tray with cooking oil.
2. Place ¾ cup white flour, all wholemeal flour, sugar, bi-carb soda, baking powder and mixed spice into a mixing bowl.
3. Lightly rub in margarine.
4. Add apple and 100ml (3fl oz) milk and lightly mix to form a soft dough.
5. Sprinkle remaining flour onto a board or bench top, turn out dough and knead gently.
6. Pat flat and cut out scones using a 6-centimetre round cutter.
7. Brush tops with remaining milk and sprinkle with cinnamon.
8. Place in oven and bake for 10 minutes or until lightly browned.

Nutrition data per scone:
478 kJ (114 cal), carbohydrate 18g, protein 3g, fat 3g, saturated fat 0.6g, fibre 2g, sodium 160mg
GI rating: low

Apricot rock cakes

Makes 16 (1 cake per serve)
Preparation/cooking time:
30 minutes

½ cup chopped dried apricots
½ cup boiling water
1½ cups self-raising flour
4 tablespoons margarine
1 tablespoon soft brown sugar
1 teaspoon ground cinnamon
¾ cup raw oats
1 egg, lightly beaten
3 tablespoons low-fat milk
2 teaspoons white sugar

Method

1. Preheat oven to 180°C (350°F) and place a sheet of baking paper on each of two flat biscuit trays.
2. Soak apricots in boiling water while you prepare the rest of the ingredients.
3. Place flour in mixing bowl and rub in margarine.
4. Add brown sugar, cinnamon and oats and mix evenly.
5. Add egg, apricots (including any liquid remaining from soaking) and milk.
6. Mix well and using two soup spoons, place spoonfuls of mixture onto biscuit trays. Allow a rounded spoonful per rock cake; 16 in total.
7. Slightly flatten and tidy edges with back of fork and sprinkle each with a little white sugar.
8. Bake for 15 minutes or until lightly browned.

Variation

Replace apricots with 1 large apple, cored, peeled and diced and add two extra tablespoons of milk to the recipe.

Nutrition data per cake:
470 kJ (112 cal), carbohydrate 14g, protein 3g, fat 4g, saturated fat 0.8g, fibre 2g, sodium 115mg
GI rating: med

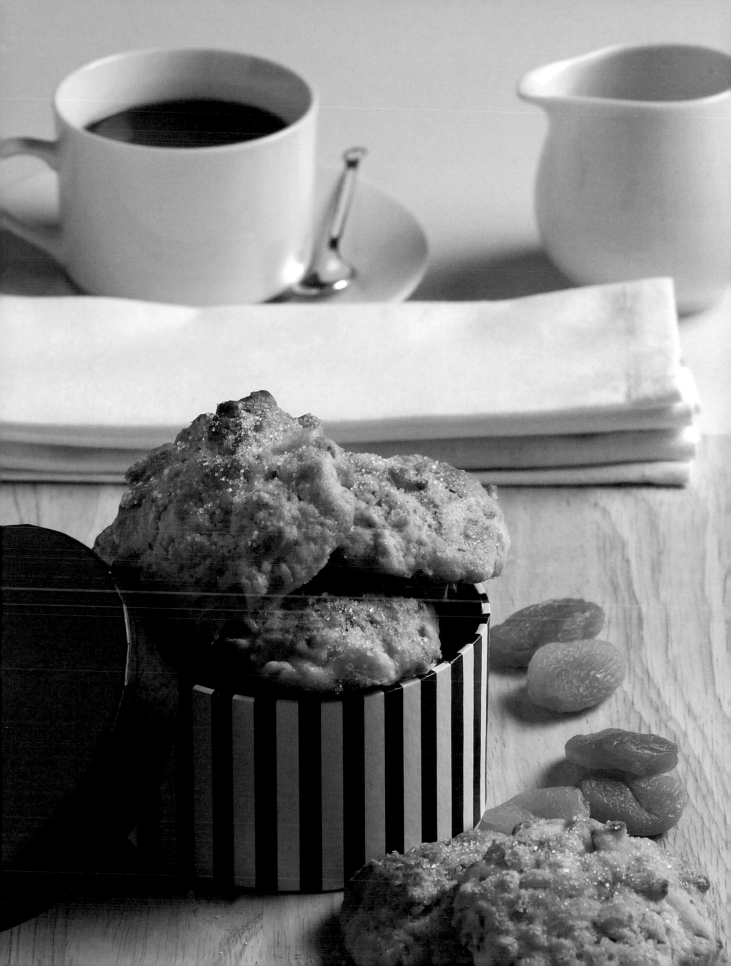

Chicken spread

Makes 2 cups (1 serve = ¼ cup)
Preparation/cooking time:
15 minutes

1 cup chopped cooked,
skinless chicken

½ cup chopped almonds or walnuts

Juice of ½ lemon

3 tablespoons low-fat natural yoghurt

Pinch mustard powder or ½ teaspoon
prepared mild mustard

1 tablespoon chopped onion

1 tablespoon chopped parsley

Method

1. Blend all ingredients and refrigerate until ready to serve.
2. Serve as a snack or light meal on triangles of wholegrain toast, use as a sandwich filling, or roll in lettuce to make parcels.
3. Cover and refrigerate any leftover spread for up to two days.

Nutrition data per serve:
372kJ (89cal), carbohydrate 1g, protein 7g, fat 6g,
saturated fat 0.7g, fibre 1g, sodium 22mg

Asparagus rolls

Serves 4 (2 per serve)
Preparation/cooking time:
10 minutes

8 slices wholegrain or low GI
white bread

8 spears asparagus—use either
fresh asparagus cooked until tender,
or use canned, drained asparagus

Low-fat mayonnaise to spread
on bread

Pepper to taste

Method

1. Cut off the crusts, roll the bread to flatten it a little, spread very lightly with low-fat mayonnaise.
2. Place a spear of asparagus diagonally across each slice of bread. Roll the bread towards the opposite corner, press lightly to seal the edges of the bread.
3. Garnish with rings of green or red capsicum and chopped parsley.
4. Serve as a snack or light meal.

Nutrition data per serve:
735 kJ (175 cal), carbohydrate 24g, protein 5g, fat 5g,
saturated fat 1.1g, fibre 4g, sodium 452mg
GI rating: low

Toast

Another great way to enjoy bread is by toasting it. This is especially good in the colder months when bread just doesn't seem as appealing.

Savoury cheese toast

Serves 4
Preparation/cooking time:
15 minutes

2 eggs

2 thin slices lean ham, chopped

90g (3oz) low-fat tasty
or block cheese, grated

1 small firm tomato, finely chopped

½ teaspoon chopped chives

Freshly ground black pepper

4 slices of wholegrain bread

Method

1. Preheat grill.
2. Place eggs in a bowl and beat lightly with a fork.
3. Add remaining ingredients, (except bread), and mix together.
4. Toast bread on one side, remove from the grill and spread the cheese mixture over the un-toasted side of the bread.
5. Grill until the mixture puffs up and browns. Serve hot as a snack or light meal.

Nutrition data per serve:
644 kJ (154 cal), carbohydrate 10g, protein 15g, fat 5g, saturated fat 2.1g, fibre 2g, sodium 463mg
GI rating: low

Lunches and light meals

Many of these light meal ideas especially foods like pizza, pasties and jacket potatoes make good foods for children and teenage parties.

The midday meal can be the main meal of the day or a lighter meal. We frequently hear the complaint 'lunches are boring—I need some ideas'. In this section we give you ideas to make your light meals more interesting, varied and lower GI. Most of the recipes in this section are useful sources of carbohydrate although some may need to be accompanied by bread or another good carbohydrate source.

Soups

Soups help satisfy hunger and can be served as an entree to a main meal or as a lunch or light meal. They can also be served as a snack after school or for the athlete, before or after training. In many instances additional carbohydrate foods should accompany the soup.

Soups can be a useful source of vegetables and carbohydrate

Soups can be useful as a source of vegetables, either as pieces or pureed to a smooth liquid. Pureed soups are a great way to disguise vegetables for those not keen on eating them. They can be made from fresh or frozen vegetables.

Most of the soups included here provide a good source of carbohydrate but in many instances additional carbohydrate foods such as a bread roll, toast or sandwich should accompany the soup. Check the carbohydrate value shown for the recipe.

Many different ingredients can be used to make soups. Some soups are thick and hearty, others thin and light. Some soups need long, slow cooking to develop the flavours, while others are very quick and easy to prepare.

The flavour of a soup often relies on the stock used in its preparation. It is easy and cheap to prepare your own stock but good pre-prepared stocks are available at most supermarkets. Alternatively, stock cubes can be successfully used although they will not give the same quality of flavour as liquid stock and tend to be high in salt. Use 1 stock cube to a cup of water.

Storage:
- Stocks can be prepared ahead of time and stored in the refrigerator or freezer for later use.
- Soups may be kept covered and refrigerated, for up to three days.
- Almost all soups freeze well so think about preparing a larger quantity than you plan to eat immediately.

Basic homemade chicken stock

Chicken stock is very useful to have on hand. It is superior to soup cubes or packet soups and we use it in many recipes. Once strained, it will keep in a sealed container in the refrigerator for up to two weeks if it is re-boiled every few days. Alternatively, freeze in bulk or in an ice cube tray and store cubes in a freezer bag for convenience.

Makes 4 cups

2 medium onions, peeled

1 large carrot

2 sticks celery

1½ kg boiling fowl

8 peppercorns

2 bay leaves

Sprig of fresh thyme
or ½ teaspoon dried thyme

5 sprigs parsley

6 cups (1½ litres) water

Salt to taste

Method:

1. Wash and roughly chop the vegetables.
2. Place all the ingredients in a large saucepan.
3. Over medium heat, slowly bring mixture to the boil. Skim off any scum that rises to the surface. Reduce heat, cover saucepan and simmer gently for three hours.
4. Strain the soup through a sieve. Reserve chicken meat for sandwiches.
5. Discard bones and vegetables.
6. Chill in refrigerator overnight and then skim off any congealed fat.

Nutritional data per serve:
Negligible

Pea, **spinach** and **chicken soup**

Serves 4
Preparation/cooking time:
45 minutes

2 cups frozen peas

3 cups Basic homemade chicken stock (page 89)

250g (8¾oz) packet frozen spinach

1 cup finely chopped, cooked chicken

2 teaspoons curry powder

Method

1. Bring stock to boil in saucepan, add frozen peas, return to the boil, and simmer until peas are tender (approximately 4–5 minutes).

2. Process stock and peas in food processor until peas are partly broken down, then return to saucepan.

3. Add spinach and simmer until the spinach is thoroughly heated (approximately 10 minutes).

4. Add chicken and curry powder; bring to the boil and serve.

Nutrition data per serve:
567 kJ (136 cal), carbohydrate 7g, protein 16g, fat 3g, saturated fat 0.7g, fibre 8g, sodium 90mg
GI rating: low

Lunches and light meals

Green pea soup

Serves 4
Preparation/cooking time:
approximately 1 hour 30 minutes

1 cup green split peas

1½ litres (6 cups) cold water

100g (3½oz) lean ham or bacon (the eye of the bacon is lower in fat), chopped

¼ cup chopped coriander or mint

2 medium carrots, peeled and grated

2 sticks celery, chopped finely

1 leek, rinsed and cut into thin rings

Pepper and salt (optional) to taste

Chopped mint to serve

Method

1. Place water, split peas, ham or bacon, and the mint or coriander in a large saucepan, bring to the boil, then simmer with the lid on until the peas are tender—they should be mostly broken up into a puree at this stage.

2. Add the vegetables, pepper and salt if needed, and bring to the boil again, Then simmer until the vegetables are tender.

3. Serve with chopped mint as a garnish.

Nutrition data per serve:
901 kJ (215 cal), carbohydrate 27g, protein 17g, fat 3g, saturated fat 0.6g, fibre 7g, sodium 425mg
GI rating: low

Old fashioned veggie soup

The barley in this soup is an excellent source of low GI carbohydrate.

Serves 4
Preparation/cooking time:
approximately 2 hours

1½ litres (6 cups) cold water

1 lamb shank, trimmed of any visible fat

½ cup pearl barley, rinsed

2 bay leaves, optional

2 sticks celery, chopped finely

2 medium carrots, peeled and grated

1 parsnip, peeled and grated

1 teaspoon dried mixed herbs

2 teaspoons beef stock powder

2 tablespoons chopped parsley to serve

Method

1. Add the water, shank, and barley to a large saucepan, bring to the boil, then simmer with lid on until meat is tender and barley soft.
2. Remove meat, cool a little, trim off any gristle and fat, chop the meat finely and return this to the saucepan.
3. Add the vegetables, prepared as above (this can be done while the shank and barley are cooking), the stock powder, and the dried herbs.
4. Simmer for about 30 minutes, until the vegetables are tender.
5. Check the flavour, adding pepper if needed. If the soup looks too thick, you can add more water—this is a very thick hearty soup though, so don't add too much!
6. Serve with parsley sprinkled over the top.

Nutrition data per serve:
711 kJ (170 cal), carbohydrate 20g, protein 11g, fat 4g, saturated fat 1.7g, fibre 5g, sodium 443mg
GI rating: low

Minestrone

There are countless versions of this hearty soup. This one has the key ingredients of the classic minestrone but is fairly quick and easy to make. It makes a satisfying lunch with a wholegrain roll. A great way to add low GI carbohydrate to your meal plan!

Serves 4
Preparation/cooking time:
1 hour

2 teaspoons olive oil

1 medium onion, peeled and chopped

1 medium carrot, peeled and sliced or chopped

2 sticks celery, washed and chopped

½ capsicum, chopped

1 medium potato, peeled and cut into dice

1 cup green beans, ends removed, and cut into 1cm lengths

1 cup shredded cabbage

4 large tomatoes, chopped

2 teaspoons olive oil

½ cup dried haricot or cannelloni beans, OR 1 can (400g/14oz) 3-bean mix or cannelloni beans, drained and rinsed

5 cups Basic homemade chicken stock (page 89)

2 bay leaves

Salt (optional) and pepper to taste

2 teaspoons dried mixed herbs

1 cup raw pasta shells, penne, or spirals

Fresh or dried parsley, grated parmesan cheese (optional) to garnish

Method

1. Heat oil in saucepan.
2. Add onion and cook, stirring, until lightly browned.
3. Add carrot, celery, capsicum and potatoes, cook for a few minutes.
4. Add dried beans (if using), cabbage, tomatoes, stock, and herbs.
5. Simmer with lid on until dried beans are cooked.
6. Add pasta, green beans, canned beans (if using), cook until pasta is cooked through. Check flavour and add salt and/or pepper to taste.
7. Serve garnished with dried or fresh chopped parsley, a sprinkle of grated parmesan cheese, and wholegrain bread or rolls.

Nutrition data per serve:
1233 kJ (295 cal), carbohydrate 46g, protein 14g, fat 4g, saturated fat 0.5g, fibre 12g, sodium 49mg
GI rating: low

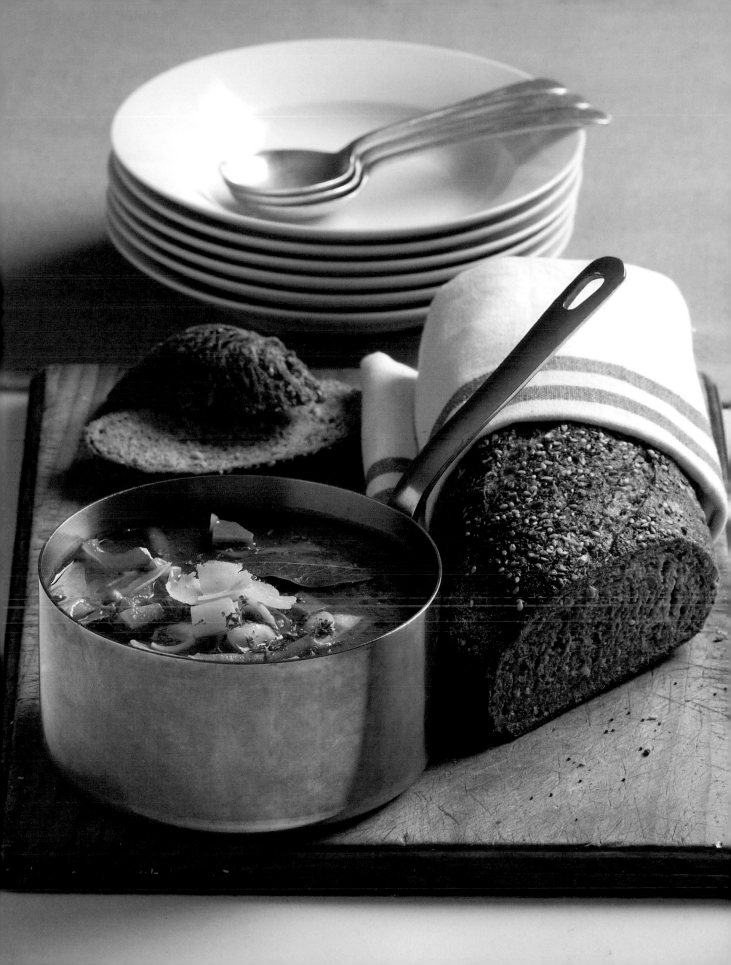

Middle Eastern lentil soup

Serves 4
Preparation/cooking time: 1 hour 20 minutes

1 cup red lentils

2 teaspoons olive oil

1 Spanish (red) onion, finely chopped OR 1 leek, sliced into rings

2 cloves garlic, crushed

1 teaspoon ground coriander

1 teaspoon ground cumin

1 teaspoon curry powder OR omit cumin and coriander and use 2 teaspoons curry powder

1 large or 2 medium carrots, peeled and grated

1 medium orange sweet potato, peeled and grated

1 tomato, finely chopped

4 cups vegetable or chicken stock

1 teaspoon grated fresh ginger

1 tablespoon lemon juice

Freshly ground black pepper

Salt to taste (optional)

3–4 tablespoons chopped fresh coriander

Method

1. Rinse the lentils and set aside.
2. Add the oil to a large saucepan and heat.
3. Add the onion, garlic and ground spices and cook, stirring, until the onion is clear.
4. Add the carrot, sweet potato, tomato, lentils, ginger and stock.
5. Bring to the boil, then reduce the heat and simmer until the vegetables are tender and the lentils soft.
6. Add the lemon juice, check the flavour and add ground black pepper and salt to taste.
7. Stir in the fresh coriander and serve.

Nutrition data per serve:
1073 kJ (257 cal), carbohydrate 37g, protein 15g, fat 4g, saturated fat 0.6g, fibre 10g, sodium 400mg
GI rating: low

Chinese chicken and **sweetcorn** soup

Serves 4
Preparation/cooking time:
45 minutes

2 teaspoons oil

2 skinless chicken fillets, finely sliced

2 cloves garlic, crushed or 1 teaspoon minced garlic

1 teaspoon chopped or grated fresh ginger

1 cup frozen corn kernels or salt-reduced canned corn kernels

4 cups Basic homemade chicken stock (page 89)

425g (15oz) can creamed sweetcorn

1 egg, lightly beaten

3 spring onions, for garnish

Method

1. Place oil in saucepan and heat until moderately hot.
2. Lightly brown sliced chicken, garlic and ginger—don't overcook.
3. Add frozen corn and stock and bring to boil.
4. Add creamed corn and simmer for 10 minutes.
5. Remove from heat when ready to serve, quickly stir in egg to make long strands.
6. Garnish with chopped spring onions.

Storage: Keeps, covered and refrigerated, for up to three days.

Nutrition data per serve:
1270 kJ (304 cal), carbohydrate 28g, protein 21g, fat 11g, saturated fat 2.7g, fibre 6g, sodium 396mg
GI rating: med

Pumpkin and sweet potato soup

Serves 4
Preparation/cooking time:
1 hour

500g (1lb) pumpkin, peeled
and cut into pieces

500g (1lb) sweet potato, orange,
peeled and cut into pieces

1 large or 2 medium onions,
peeled and chopped

2 teaspoons margarine

1 teaspoon oil

1–2 teaspoons curry powder

1 teaspoon ground cumin

1 teaspoon ground coriander

1 teaspoon ground nutmeg

pepper to taste

1 litre (4 cups) homemade
basic stock

Method

1. Add margarine and oil to large saucepan and heat until melted (oil is used to prevent margarine from burning).
2. Add dry spices except nutmeg and stir over the heat for about 1 minute—don't allow to burn.
3. Add the onion and brown lightly, stirring to avoid burning.
4. Add the pumpkin and sweet potato, stock, and the nutmeg, bring to the boil, then simmer until the pumpkin and sweet potato are tender.
5. Process until smooth, check the flavour, adding pepper if desired.
6. Serve with a grainy roll, wholegrain toast, or a savoury low GI muffin.

Optional: chopped fresh coriander or parsley can be sprinkled on top when serving.

Nutrition data per serve:
744 kJ (178 cal), carbohydrate 29g, protein 6g, fat 4g, saturated fat 0.9g, fibre 5g, sodium 32mg
GI rating: low

Sandwiches, toast and bread ideas

Ideas for sandwiches are endless. Choose low GI bread (look for the symbol on the packet) such as pumpernickel, wholegrain rye and wheat, soy and linseed, oats and barley, genuine sour dough bread and white breads displaying the GI symbol. The filling in sandwiches should provide the texture and flavour and there is usually no need to spread the bread with butter or margarine. Many of these sandwiches can be toasted.

Fillings:

The following list of ideas might help you get started with delicious sandwich fillings to keep lunchtime boredom away. Remember when you use any of these fillings you do not need to use margarine on the bread. Most fillings can be used for traditional sandwiches, for jaffles or toasted sandwiches, for wraps, or for open sandwiches.

Cheese and....

- grated low-fat tasty or block cheese, grated apple, carrot, chopped celery and pecans or walnuts mixed with low-fat cream cheese
- low-fat ricotta cheese with sliced cucumber, tomato, chopped basil and a grinding of pepper
- low-fat ricotta cheese with chopped celery and walnuts
- grated low-fat tasty or block cheese, mustard and sun-dried tomatoes
- sliced low-fat tasty or block cheese, thinly sliced green apple and fruit chutney
- low-fat cream cheese or low-fat mayonnaise and asparagus
- cottage cheese with chopped pineapple and sultanas or chopped or flaked almonds.

Fish and....

- salmon or tuna (drained) with sliced cucumber or celery, topped with low-fat mayonnaise
- prawn, low-fat ricotta cheese and thinly sliced cucumber
- smoked salmon, low-fat cream cheese and capers
- salmon or tuna (drained), mixed with a little curry powder, lemon juice, parsley, and low-fat mayonnaise or coleslaw dressing
- salmon or tuna (drained) mixed with low-fat mayonnaise and some sweet chilli sauce and slices of tomato
- sardines with thinly sliced onion, a squeeze of lemon, and freshly ground pepper.

Meat or chicken and....
- thinly sliced cold lean meat topped with mango chutney or mustard
- chopped chicken, chives and parsley mixed with low-fat mayonnaise and shredded lettuce
- chopped chicken, walnuts and celery or green capsicum mixed with low-fat natural yoghurt
- chopped lean ham, whole seed mustard, and grated apple
- chopped chicken topped with thinly sliced raw mushrooms and fruit chutney
- cold lean roast lamb with mint jelly, tomato, and lettuce
- chicken spread (see page 86) with sliced tomato and cucumber.

Egg and....
- scrambled eggs with finely chopped lean ham
- hard-boiled eggs mashed with alfalfa or bean sprouts, low-fat mayonnaise and curry powder
- sliced hard boiled egg with grated carrot and gherkin spread.

Vegetables and....
- canned baked beans, lightly mashed and seasoned with tabasco sauce
- peanut butter and sliced cucumber or chopped celery
- mashed kidney or three-bean mix with sweet chilli sauce or mild salsa, capsicum, cucumber and onion
- crushed peanuts with grated carrot and alfalfa sprouts.

Sweet fillings and....
- mashed banana, lemon juice and cinnamon
- cottage or low-fat ricotta cheese with chopped dried fig
- peanut butter and honey.

Bruschettas

This is simply a style of making toast that involves toasting thickly cut bread, spreading it with a little olive oil and perhaps rubbing it lightly with a clove of freshly peeled garlic, then toasting lightly again to bring out the oil and garlic aromas and flavours. You can then add a topping and serve either hot or cold for a quick and tasty lunch or light meal or with a drink or as an entrée.

Note:
Bruschettas do need to be prepared just before serving, otherwise the bread becomes soggy.

Mushroom and herb bruschetta

Serves 4 (2 slices per serve)
Preparation/cooking time:
20 minutes

300g (10½oz) mushrooms, sliced

6 spring onions, trimmed
and sliced finely

Rind of 1 lemon, grated

½ cup chopped parsley

2 tablespoons chives, chopped

Pepper and salt (optional) to taste

8 slices thickly cut grainy
or sour dough bread

1 tablespoon olive oil
or olive oil spray

2 cloves garlic, freshly peeled

125g (4½oz) low-fat cream cheese
(80% fat reduced)

Method

1. Spray a small frying pan with oil and heat.
2. Add the mushrooms, onions, lemon rind, parsley and chives, pepper and salt, and cook until the mushrooms start to brown and the liquid evaporates.
3. Toast or grill the bread. While still warm, drizzle or spray oil over and rub with the garlic (using olive oil spray lightly will lower the fat content).
4. Place the bread under the grill again until hot, remove and put onto plates to serve.
5. Spread each toast slice with cream cheese, top with the mushroom mixture, and serve while warm.

Nutrition data per serve:
1183 kJ (283 cal), carbohydrate 27g, protein 10g, fat 14g, saturated fat 4.6g, fibre 5g, sodium 400mg
GI rating: low

Tomato and basil bruschetta

Serves 4 (2 slices per serve)
Preparation/cooking time:
15 minutes

3 large tomatoes, chopped into small chunks

100g (3½oz) semi-dried tomatoes, well drained

½ cup basil leaves, chopped

Pepper and salt (optional) to taste

1 large red onion, peeled, chopped finely

2 teaspoons balsamic vinegar

1 teaspoon sugar

8 slices thickly cut grainy or sour dough bread

1 tablespoon olive oil

1–2 cloves garlic, freshly peeled

2 tablespoons tomato paste

garnish—a little chopped basil

Method

1. Place fresh tomatoes in a strainer to remove excess water then combine with the basil, pepper and salt, onion, vinegar and sugar, set aside.
2. Toast or grill the bread. While still warm, drizzle oil over and rub with the garlic. (You can replace the drizzled oil with a light spray of olive oil spray).
3. Place the bread under the grill again until hot, remove and put onto plates to serve.
4. Spread the bread with tomato paste, pile the tomato topping on the bread, and garnish with a little of the chopped basil.

Nutrition data per serve:
1197 kJ (286 cal), carbohydrate 40g, protein 10g, fat 7g, saturated fat 1.0g, fibre 9g, sodium 384mg
GI rating: low

Hamburgers in grainy rolls

These hamburgers are simple. If you like, you can spread the rolls with tomato or steak sauce,
or a light mayonnaise and/or add other vegetables, such as sliced onion or beetroot.

Serves 4
(1 hamburger per serve)
Preparation/cooking time:
30 minutes

½ quantity of rissole mixture
(see page 187)

4 lettuce leaves, washed

2 tomatoes, sliced thinly

4 grainy rolls

Method

1. Make rissoles and cook (see rissole recipe).

2. While rissoles are cooking, split rolls and toast the cut sides.

3. Prepare the tomatoes and lettuce.

4. When the rissoles are cooked, place 1 rissole on each roll, place 2–3 tomato slices on top, cover with a lettuce leaf and serve.

Nutrition data per serve:
1265 kJ (303 cal), carbohydrate 34g, protein 20g, fat 8g, saturated fat 2.3g, fibre 6g, sodium 390mg
GI rating: low

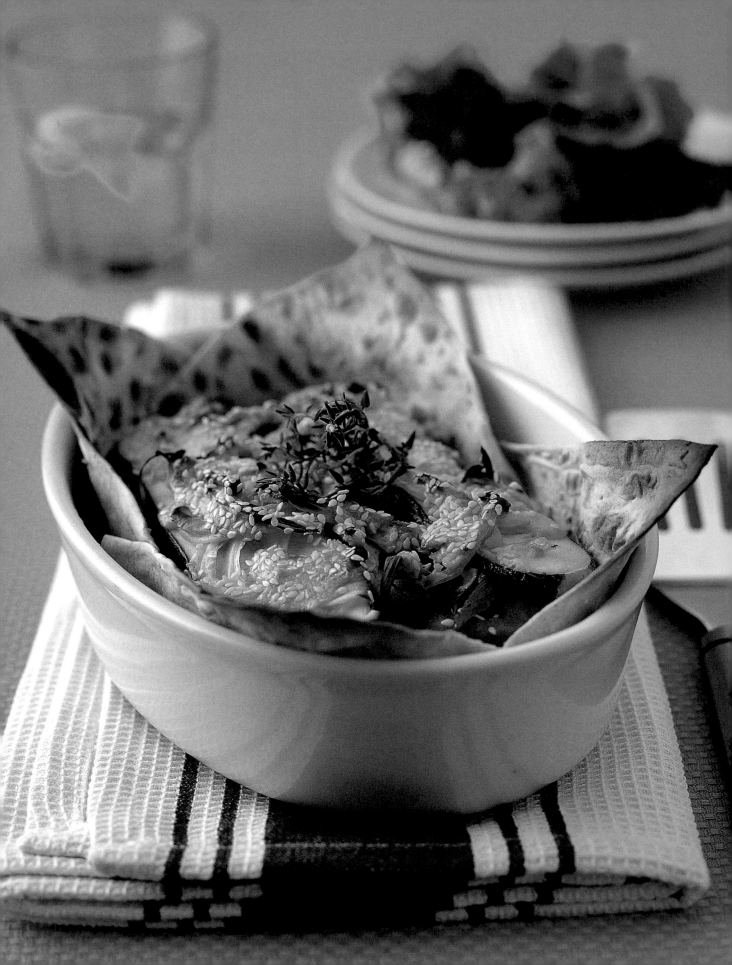

Zucchini and tomato lavash bake

Serves 4
Preparation/cooking time:
1 hour

2 teaspoons margarine or oil

2 rounds of lavash bread

2 medium zucchini, cut in half crossways, and then into strips

3 tomatoes, sliced

4 spring onions, chopped

2 teaspoons fresh herbs, chopped, or 1 teaspoon dried mixed herbs

Pinch salt (optional) and pepper

1 medium onion, sliced

1 tablespoon tahini

Juice of ½ lemon

¼ teaspoon finely chopped or minced fresh ginger

¼ teaspoon prepared mustard

2 tablespoons sesame seeds

Method

1. Preheat oven to 200ºC (400ºF)
2. Spread margarine or oil over a casserole dish.
3. Place bread in casserole. Push into corners without breaking it, and leave excess hanging out.
4. Place half of the zucchini in the bottom.
5. Cover with the sliced tomato.
6. Sprinkle spring onions, herbs, salt and pepper over (if using).
7. Add the remainder of the zucchini, then the finely sliced onion.
8. Blend tahini, lemon juice, ginger, mustard and a little water to make a thin paste and pour over vegetables.
9. Sprinkle with sesame seeds.
10. Fold edges of bread in around the edge of the casserole to form a crust around the edge and over the top.
11. Bake in oven for 40–45 minutes or until the bread is brown and crusty, and the zucchini is tender.

Nutrition data per serve:
869 kJ (208 cal), carbohydrate 23g, protein 7g, fat 9g, saturated
fat 1.2g, fibre 5g, sodium 186mg
GI rating: med

Pizzas

Commercial pizzas are often quite high in fat. Making a pizza at home is easy, so why not try some of our quick and tasty ideas? Pizza is particularly good as a light meal in cold weather when looking for something hot.

You can purchase fresh or frozen pizza bases in the supermarket, but they will generally be high GI. There are alternatives you can use to make absolutely delicious pizzas for lunch or a light meal.

Wholegrain pita bread (see recipe below) and Wholegrain English muffins both make suitable pizza bases.

Sauces

- Tomato paste—thin with a little water, add some fresh or dried mixed herbs
- Pizza sauce—available from supermarkets
- Tomato-based pasta sauce
- Pesto—high in fat so use sparingly

Toppings

- Meat: lean ham, chopped chicken, leftover roast, bolognese sauce (see page 138).
- Fish: canned tuna or salmon, smoked salmon, prawns
- Vegetables: onion, capsicum, zucchini slices, corn, tomato slices, mushrooms, sun-dried tomatoes, cooked broccoli florets, spring onion, snow peas, fresh spinach leaves, asparagus, cooked cold vegetables—potato, pumpkin, sweet potato—whatever you have!
- Cheese: low-fat cheeses do not melt well, so there are some other options:
  -try light mozzarella (available in supermarkets already grated, and lower in fat than the regular mozzarella—and it does freeze for later use)
  - use cut up boccochini or crumbled low-fat feta cheese rather than melting cheese
  - a little freshly grated parmesan—this is a high fat cheese, but if you use it sparingly, the end result will be fairly low in fat

Cheese is actually not essential for a pizza—using tasty sauces, fresh and dried herbs, and flavoursome ingredients will give a pizza plenty of taste!

Quick muffin pizzas

Serves 4 (1 muffin per serve)
Preparation/cooking time:
20 minutes

4 wholegrain English muffins—
buy grainy ones if possible

2 tablespoons low-salt
tomato paste

½ cup chopped cooked chicken
or 2 slices lean ham, chopped;
or 1 small can tuna or salmon

1 tomato, sliced thinly

2 mushrooms, sliced

½ capsicum, sliced thinly

1 small onion, sliced thinly

Other toppings as available,
for example, cooked vegetables,
snow peas, zucchini slices

¾ cup grated low-fat
mozzarella cheese

Method

1. Preheat oven to 200°C (400°F), or light griller
2. Split the muffins and place on a tray.
3. Spread some sauce thinly over each half muffin—so they don't become soggy.
4. Add toppings—try different combinations.
5. Sprinkle cheese over.
6. Place in oven or under griller until the cheese is melted and starting to brown a little.
7. Serve while still hot—although cold leftover pizza also makes a great snack any time of day!

Nutrition data per serve:
1119 kJ (268 cal), carbohydrate 26g, protein 19g, fat 9g, saturated fat 4.2g, fibre 5g, sodium 368mg
GI rating: low

Pita pizza

The beauty of this recipe is that by using pita bread as the pizza base, you can put the whole dish together very quickly, which makes it an ideal snack or light meal. The pizzas also freeze well.

**Serves 4
(1 pita bread per serve)
Preparation/cooking time:
30 minutes**

4 small wholegrain pita breads

½ cup commercial pasta sauce,
no added salt, tomato-based

3 large tomatoes, sliced

1 medium green capsicum,
de-seeded and sliced

1 cup sliced mushrooms

1 medium onion, peeled and sliced

8 tablespoons grated,
low-fat tasty or block cheese

16 black olives, chopped
(optional)

1 zucchini sliced (optional)

Method

1. Preheat oven to 180°C (350ºF)

2. Spread pita breads with sauce. Arrange the vegetables evenly over the top and sprinkle with grated cheese.

3. Place on a baking tray. Bake in oven for 15–20 minutes or until cheese melts and begins to brown.

4. Serve pita pizzas straight from the oven, accompanied by a tossed salad.

Storage: Wrap prepared but uncooked pizzas in plastic film or slide into big freezer bags and freeze until needed, then place the frozen pizzas on a baking tray and bake up to 25 minutes or until golden brown.

Nutrition data per serve:
1034 kJ (247 cal), carbohydrate 35g, protein 15g, fat 4g, saturated fat 1.3g, fibre 6g, sodium 396mg
GI rating: med

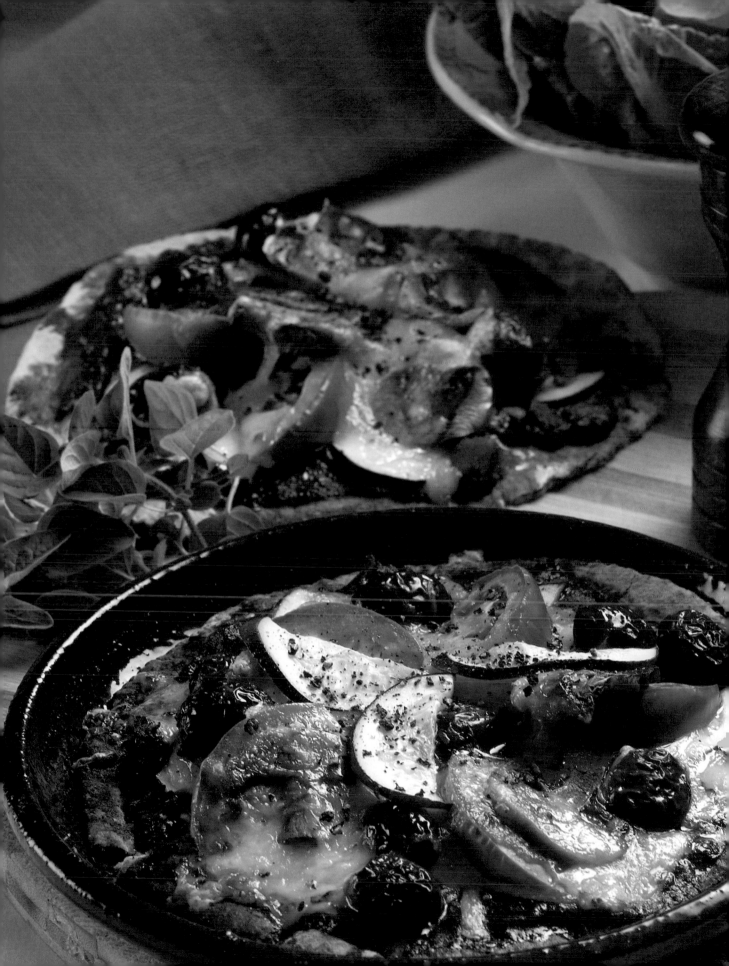

Pastry

The fillings used in pastry dishes can help reduce the GI of a dish

Quiche can be a tasty alternative to a bread-based meal. Although most pastry is high GI, the fillings can overcome this effect, especially if low GI vegetables and milk form the basis of the filling.

Quick and easy 'all-in-one' quiche

This quiche makes its own crust! It is so quick and easy to make, and is delicious hot or cold served with crusty bread and a green salad.

Serves 4
Preparation/cooking time:
1 hour

4 eggs

1 cup skim milk

1 cup full-cream natural yoghurt

2 tablespoons wholemeal plain flour

1 cup low-fat ricotta cheese

½ cup chopped spring onions

120g (4oz) mushrooms, sliced

1 medium tomato, diced

Spray oil

330g (11oz) can asparagus, drained

Method

1. Preheat oven to 180°C (350°F)
2. Beat together eggs, milk, yoghurt and flour.
3. Add cheese, spring onions, mushrooms and tomato.
4. Pour into a lightly oiled flan dish.
5. Arrange asparagus on top.
6. Bake in oven for 30–35 minutes or until quiche is set and lightly browned.

Storage: Keeps in the refrigerator for up to three days.

Nutrition data per serve:
1218 kJ (291 cal), carbohydrate 17g, protein 23g, fat 13g, saturated fat 6g, fibre 5g, sodium 371mg
GI rating: low

Pasties

Makes 12 (1 shortcrust pastie or 2 filo pasties per serve)
Preparation/cooking time: 1 hour

200g (7oz) lean minced beef

2 medium potatoes, washed, finely diced

1 large carrot, finely diced

1 small or ½ medium swede, finely diced

1 large onion, finely diced

¼ teaspoon white pepper

Salt to taste (optional)

1 teaspoon dried mixed herbs

4 tablespoons finely chopped parsley

3 sheets shortcrust pastry
OR 12 sheets filo pastry

1 tablespoon water

Spray oil

Nutrition data per serve (shortcrust)
1064 kJ (254 cal), carbohydrate 25g, protein 8g, fat 13g, saturated fat 6.5g, fibre 3g, sodium 200mg
GI rating: med

If served with asparagus and bean salad the fibre content per serve will increase to 6 grams.

Nutrition data per serve (filo)
892 kJ (213 cal), carbohydrate 29g, protein 13g, fat 4g, saturated fat 1.2g, fibre 5g, sodium 248mg
GI rating: med

Method

1. Preheat oven to 200°C (400°F)
2. Place potato, swede, and carrot in a microwave oven dish and cook until just tender (about 4 minutes). This shortens final cooking time.
3. In a bowl, combine meat, diced cooked vegetables, onion, seasonings and herbs.
4. On a lightly floured board, roll out each sheet of shortcrust pastry to make a slightly larger sheet. Divide into four equal portions.
5. Divide the meat mixture between the pastry squares, placing a good spoonful on one side.
6. Brush the edges of the pastry with a little water.
7. Fold pastry over in half, to make a pasty—this makes a triangle shape.
8. Use the back of a fork to crimp the edges of the pasties firmly.
9. Repeat with each sheet of pastry.
10. Place the finished pasties on a lightly greased baking tray.
11. Prick the top of each pasty three times with a fork.
12. Spray with a little oil.
13. Bake in oven for 35 minutes or until browned.
14. Serve with Asparagus and green bean salad (page 206).

If using filo pastry: At step 3, place 1 sheet filo on a clean bench, spray lightly with oil, cover with the second sheet, spray this also with oil, then place the third sheet over the top.

Cut in half so you have 2 squares of pastry. Place some filling near one edge and fold into a parcel, making sure you slightly wet the last edge before folding over—this keeps the pastry together. Place, edge side down, on a baking sheet. Spray with oil. Repeat process until you have 12 pasty 'parcels'. Bake as above.

Storage: Freeze uncooked pasties in freezer bags or other suitable container. Defrost shortcrust pasties before baking (re-heat pasties made with filo pastry from the frozen state).

Mushroom stroganoff

This makes a tasty topping for bruschetta or jacket potatoes, or as a sauce for grilled meat.

Serves 4
Preparation/cooking time:
15 minutes

Spray oil

2 onions, sliced

1 red or green capsicum, diced

16–20 medium-sized button
mushrooms, sliced

1 teaspoon paprika

Sprinkle lemon pepper
or ground black pepper

1 cup low-fat, natural yoghurt

3 tablespoons chopped parsley

3 spring onions, chopped

Method

1. Spray frying pan lightly with oil.
2. Add the onions, capsicum, mushrooms, paprika and lemon pepper and allow to brown and cook down a little—stir to avoid sticking and burning. The mushrooms should be soft. Remove from heat.
3. Place yoghurt in a bowl, gradually fold in mushroom mixture.
4. Do not reheat as yoghurt will curdle.
5. Garnish with parsley and spring onions to serve.

Nutrition data per serve:
366 kJ (88 cal), carbohydrate 9g, protein 8g, fat 1g, saturated fat trace, fibre 3g, sodium 59mg
GI rating: low

Potatoes

Potatoes have a high GI, but if left whole with the skin on, as in jacket potatoes, the GI is a little lower than when potato is mashed. If you serve jacket potatoes with a salad using a dressing that includes lemon juice or vinegar, you can lower the GI of the whole meal.

Jacket potatoes

Serves 4 (1 potato per serve)
Preparation/cooking time:
15–60 minutes (depending on
cooking method for potatoes)

4 medium-sized potatoes

Method

1. Wash potatoes well, do not peel. Prick several times with a fork or skewer. For a crispy skin do not cover. For a softer skin wrap potatoes in foil.

2. Bake the potatoes in a preheated 180°C (350°F) Gas Mark 4 oven for 45–60 minutes or until tender when tested with a skewer. Alternatively, cook uncovered in the microwave on high for 6–8 minutes (depending on your microwave), turning them over halfway through cooking—check how soft they are and adjust remainder of cooking time. Prepare fillings while potatoes cook.

3. Serve plain or try some of the following delicious fillings, or a combination of your own.

Fillings (These toppings serve 4 with 1 potato per serve):

Cheesy bean topping

Split the top of each potato, spoon over ⅓ cup baked beans, top with 1 tablespoon low-fat grated cheese, and either place in the microwave oven for 1-2 minutes to heat the topping, or place under a hot griller

Nutrition data per serve:
975 kJ (233 cal), carbohydrate 37g, protein 13g, fat 1g, saturated fat 0.7g, fibre 8g, sodium 452mg
GI rating: high

Beef 'n bean
(1 potato per serve)

Split the potatoes, spoon over ¼ cup bolognese sauce (see page 138), and top with 2 tablespoons baked beans, or kidney beans or 3-bean mix.

Nutrition data per serve:
884 kJ (211 cal), carbohydrate 30g, protein 12g, fat 3g, saturated fat 1g, fibre 5g, sodium 172mg
GI rating: high

Coleslaw

Split the tops of the potatoes, spoon 1 tablespoon low-fat grated cheese onto each, and top with ½ cup coleslaw (see page 211)

Nutrition data per serve:
788 kJ (188 cal), carbohydrate 11g, protein g, fat 2g, saturated fat 0.8g, fibre 6g, sodium 203mg
GI rating: high

Mushroom stroganoff

Use ½ quantity of mushroom stroganoff (see page opposite)

Nutrition data per serve:
761 kJ (182 cal), carbohydrate 31g, protein 9g, fat 1g, saturated fat trace, fibre 6g, sodium 128mg
GI rating: high

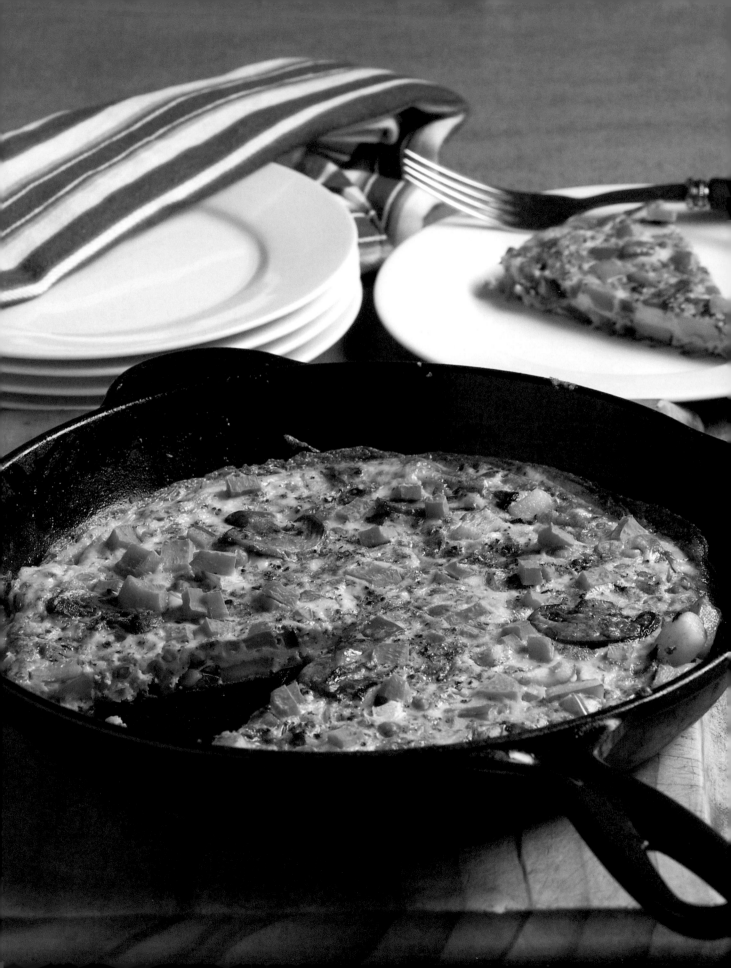

Spanish omelette

Delicious cold or hot, this omelette is a great way of using up leftover cooked and uncooked vegetables. This recipe is low in carbohydrate but it has a high GI rating. To lower the GI of this recipe use less potato and increase the other vegetables. The inclusion of eggs in this dish also helps lowers the GI

Serves 4
Preparation/cooking time:
45 minutes

1 teaspoon margarine

1 teaspoon oil

2 medium potatoes, diced but not peeled

1 large onion, chopped

6 large mushrooms, chopped

½ green or red capsicum, chopped

1 cup cooked vegetables (e.g. corn, peas, carrots, sweet potato, asparagus)

5 eggs

¼ teaspoon black pepper

¼ teaspoon ground nutmeg

1 teaspoon dried mixed herbs

Pinch salt (optional)

1 tablespoons chopped parsley

Few drops tabasco sauce or pinch cayenne pepper

¼ cup water

Method

1. Heat margarine and oil in frying pan over medium-high heat.
2. Add potato and onion. Cover and cook over low heat for approximately 10–15 minutes until potatoes are tender.
3. Add mushrooms, capsicum, cooked vegetables and cook a further five minutes.
4. Beat eggs with seasonings and water.
5. Pour over vegetables in frying pan, cover, and cook over low heat until almost set. Do not allow bottom to burn.
6. Preheat grill to medium, and slide omelette under the grill to complete cooking.
7. Loosen omelette and turn onto warm plate.
8. Cut into wedges to serve.

Storage: Cover and refrigerate for up to two days.

Nutrition data per serve:
989 kJ (237 cal), carbohydrate 23g, protein 14g, fat 9g, saturated fat 2.3g, fibre 5g, sodium 105mg
GI rating: med

High-carb salads

Salads not only make great additions to a main meal, but can 'stand alone' as a light meal or lunch, or even a snack, especially if they include plenty of lower-GI carbohydrate (such as pasta, pulses, or lower GI rice), and some protein. The recipes here give you some ideas to get you started.

Rice salad with roasted peanuts

Serves 4
Preparation/cooking time:
30 minutes

2 cups cooked Mahatma™ white, long grain or basmati rice

½ green capsicum, chopped

½ red capsicum, chopped

4 spring onions, sliced

4 radishes, finely sliced

1 stick celery, finely sliced

½ cup unsalted dry roasted peanuts

½ cup canned water chestnuts, drained and sliced

½ cup green beans, blanched

1 tablespoon light soy sauce

1 teaspoon sugar

2 tablespoons chopped parsley

½ cup bean sprouts

Pinch of salt (optional)

Method

1. Combine all ingredients.
2. Chill.
3. Serve garnished with chopped spring onions and radish slices.

Nutrition data per serve:
1078 kJ (258 cal), carbohydrate 32g, protein 9g, fat 10g, saturated fat 1g, fibre 5g, sodium 314mg
GI rating: low–med

Fettuccine salmon salad

Serves 4
Preparation/cooking time:
45 minutes

4 cups water

250g (8¾oz) fresh spinach
fettuccine

6 spring onions

½ stick celery

½ capsicum

1 tomato

½ zucchini

½ avocado

200g (7oz) can pink or red
salmon, drained, skin
and bones removed

1 cup grated carrot

Dressing:
2 tablespoons chopped mint

Juice ½ lemon

Juice 1 orange

2 teaspoons olive oil

2 teaspoons light soy sauce

Method

1. Heat water until boiling. Add fettuccine and cook until al dente (tender). Drain, rinse and cool.
2. Chop spring onions, celery, capsicum and tomato.
3. Cut zucchini into fine strips.
4. Peel avocado and roughly chop.
5. Combine pasta with vegetables and salmon, mix gently.
6. Mix mint, lemon juice, orange juice, olive oil and soy sauce.
7. Pour dressing over the salad and toss lightly.

Nutrition data per serve:
1168 kJ (279 cal), carbohydrate 23g, protein 16g, fat 13g, saturated fat 2.8g, fibre 4g, sodium 446mg
GI rating: low

Broad bean
and **smoked salmon** salad

Although the GI of this dish is rated high, the total carbohydrate per serve is small.

Serves 4
Preparation/cooking time:
20 minutes

250g (8¾oz) broad beans, frozen
or fresh

85g (3oz) smoked salmon,
thinly sliced

24 cherry tomatoes, halved

1 large red onion, thinly sliced

Dressing:
2 tablespoons lemon juice

2 teaspoons olive oil

2 teaspoons capers, drained

2 tablespoons chopped
fresh parsley

Method

1. Cook broad beans until they are soft but still retain their shape.
2. Combine broad beans, smoked salmon, cherry tomatoes and onion in a bowl.
3. Blend the dressing ingredients in a screw top jar and pour over the salad.
4. Chill and serve.

Nutrition data per serve:
522 kJ (129 cal), carbohydrate 9g, protein 11g, fat 4g, saturated fat 0.6g, fibre 5g, sodium 383mg
GI rating: med

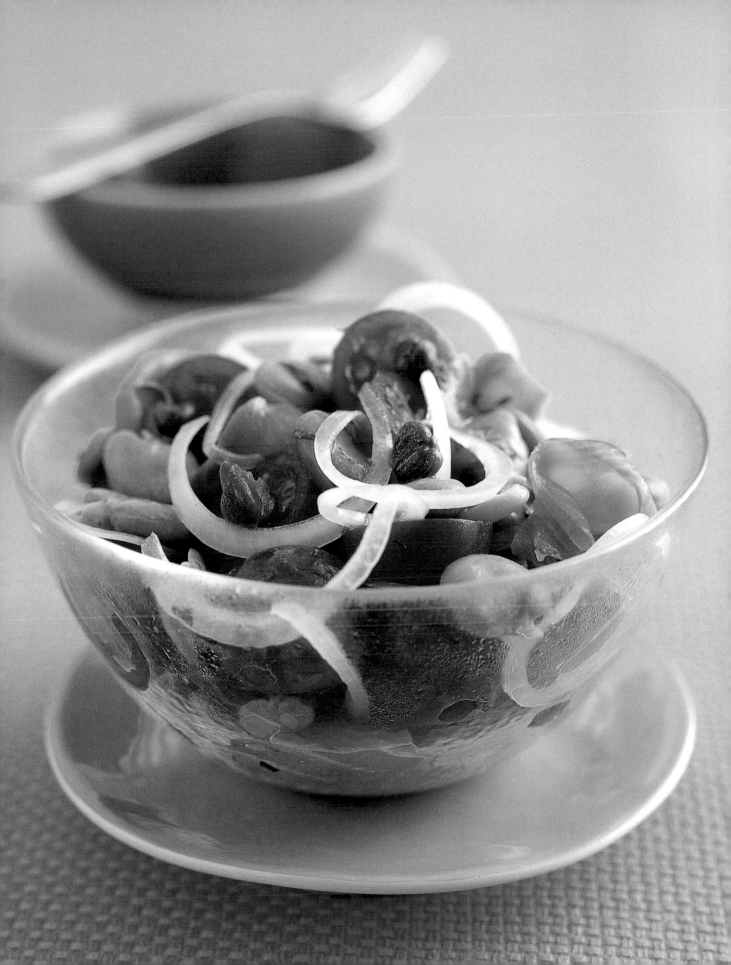

Curried pasta salad

Serves 4

Preparation/cooking time:
30 minutes

1½ cups shell pasta

4 hard-boiled eggs

½ cup diced celery

4 spring onions, chopped

2 tablespoons sultanas

½ green capsicum, diced

2 tablespoons chopped parsley

½ cup corn kernels

½ quantity curry dressing (see page 220)

Method

1. Cook pasta in boiling water for 10–12 minutes until al dente (tender), drain and then run cold water over to cool.
2. Cut eggs into quarters and combine with pasta, celery, spring onions, sultanas, capsicum, parsley and corn.
3. Spoon curry dressing over and toss.
4. Refrigerate for one hour before serving.

Nutrition data per serve:
1283 kJ (307 cal), carbohydrate 46g, protein 15g, fat 6g, saturated fat 1.6g, fibre 5g, sodium 237mg
GI rating: low

Nicoise salad

Serves 4

Preparation/cooking time: 20 minutes

8 baby potatoes (chats) cooked and cut into 4

2 eggs, hard boiled, cut into quarters

200g (7oz) can tuna chunks in water, drained and roughly flaked

1 cup green beans, trimmed, cut into 2cm (½ inch) lengths, cooked lightly

1 large red onion, peeled and sliced thinly

1 punnet (250g, 9oz) cherry tomatoes, cut into halves if larger otherwise leave whole OR 4 medium tomatoes, cut into small chunks

1 small Lebanese cucumber, cut into chunks

¼ cup black olives, pitted (optional)

Method

1. Place all the salad ingredients in a large salad bowl.
2. Combine dressing ingredients, check flavour and adjust, pour over salad and mix carefully to leave the tuna and egg in nice pieces for good presentation.

Dressing:

Juice ½ lemon

1 tablespoon olive oil

1 teaspoon sugar

½ teaspoon grated or minced garlic

Freshly grated black pepper

OR use 2–3 tablespoons low oil French dressing

Nutrition data per serve:
1083 kJ (259 cal), carbohydrate 22g, protein 20g, fat 9g, saturated fat 1.9g, fibre 5g, sodium 159mg
GI rating: high

Mixed bean salad

This salad is wonderful for a barbeque. It makes a large amount—you can halve the recipe, use the leftovers as a hot or cold dish for another meal, or top jacket potatoes with a generous spoonful of this salad for a tasty lunch.

Serves 8
Preparation/cooking time:
30 minutes

400g can (14oz) 4-bean mix, drained and rinsed

200g (7oz) can corn kernels, drained

½ cup green beans, cut into 2cm (¾in) lengths, cooked lightly —microwave is ideal

1 cup cooked pasta spirals or bows

½ red onion, peeled and thinly sliced

1 green or red capsicum, seeded and diced

2 tablespoons chopped parsley or basil

Dressing:
Juice ½ lemon

1 tablespoon olive oil

2 tablespoons balsamic vinegar

2 teaspoons prepared mild mustard—American is ideal

2 teaspoons sugar

Salt (optional) and pepper to taste

Method

1. In a large bowl, combine the drained beans, corn, green beans, pasta, onion, capsicum, and parsley.
2. Combine the dressing ingredients, check flavour and adjust to taste, pour over the salad and toss well.
3. Refrigerate until ready to serve.

Nutrition data per serve:
542 kJ (130 cal), carbohydrate 18g, protein 5g, fat 3g, saturated fat 0.4g, fibre 5g, sodium 249mg
GI rating: low

Other salads can be found on pages 206–214.

Lunches and light meals

Main meals

Plan your main meals by balancing the carbohydrate and protein foods with vegetables
Follow these steps to plan a balanced meal:

- **Choose your carbohydrate**: rice, pasta, noodles, potato, pancakes, couscous, polenta, legumes, breads, cereals. Don't forget to include at least one or two low GI carbohydrate foods at each meal.
- **Consider your protein**: meat, poultry, fish, seafood, eggs, tofu, pulses/legumes, cheese, nuts.
- **Add plenty of vegetables and maybe some fruit**: cooked or raw, as either the main part of a dish or as a side dish.
- **Choose your flavour**: traditionally, the Australian diet has been rather plain and the flavours monotonous but over recent years the influence of other cultures, in particular those of the Indian sub-continent, Asia, and the Mediterranean, has encouraged us to add interest to our meals. The variety of herbs and spices and addition of garlic, onions, ginger and chilli is common.
- **Consider the fat**: much of the fat in meals will come from the ingredients; some will be added during cooking. Remember the guideline—limit saturated fats by choosing lean or low-fat animal foods and use unsaturated fat and oils in moderation. We show you how in our recipes.

Stir-frys

The stir-fry is a good way to show how you can follow the steps in planning balanced meals.
Increasingly, many of our cooking methods and food choices are influenced by several factors:

- lack of time for food preparation
- the influence of Asian and Mediterranean cuisines
- rapidly increasing availability of prepared and semi-prepared foods in the supermarket
- a preference by many to use less meat by making it part of a dish rather than the main component.

These changes are reflected in the popularity of the stir-fry as a family meal choice, one of the easiest ways to prepare a quick, colourful and interesting meal. It can be varied to suit individual tastes and can form the basis of a vegetarian, seafood or meat meal. Just about any vegetable can be tossed in a pan or wok with a touch of oil, water or stock, garlic, herbs and spices and served with noodles or rice.

Basic stir-fry cooking

The secret of a successful stir-fry is to have all the ingredients prepared before you begin cooking, and then to cook them swiftly so that they reach the table still crisp, full of flavour, and with the colours bright and fresh looking.

Follow these steps to balanced and delicious meals:

- Choose your carbohydrate
- Consider your protein
- Add plenty of vegetables
- Choose your flavour
- Consider the fat.

Step 1: Choose your carbohydrate:

Include low GI carbohydrate in all meals and snacks to help control your blood glucose levels and satisfy your appetite.

Traditionally either rice or noodles are served with stir-fries. These add the fuel component of the dish, as most stir-fries are made with low carbohydrate vegetables.

Allow 1½ cup uncooked rice or 300g (10½oz) uncooked noodles for 4 people.

Rice

The amount of the different starch types (see page xx) contained in the different varieties of rice changes their GI rating making some better choices than others.

Most Australian grown short and long grain, white or brown rice, such as Calrose, and the sticky, glutinous and parboiled rices have high GI values.

The Australian grown long grain doongara, long grain basmati or Mahatma™ white, long grain, Japanese short grain rice and Arborio (a rice often used in risottos) have lower or medium GI's.

For rice dishes see page xx

Noodles

Noodles are like long, thin spaghetti. They cook quickly and are great added to soups or stir-fries. In many recipes they can be interchanged with rice. Most noodles are either made from wheat or rice although some are made from beans:

- vermicilli, which is wheat based also has a low GI
- instant noodles are also wheat based and are popular with many as they make a quick and filling meal or snack. Most are high in fat and the flavour sachets that accompany them high in salt and mono sodium glutamate

- rice noodles can be purchased fresh or dried. Fresh rice noodles have low GI and are usually a better choice than dried ones that have a higher GI.
- cellophane noodles, are made from mung beans and have a low GI.
- Fresh rice and wheat-based noodles have a lower GI than dried rice noodles.
- As well as being great in stir fries, you will find several recipes that use noodles in other parts of this book (see Nibbles and party foods page 248)

Step 2: Consider your protein

Allow 500g (1lb) for 4 people—any meat or fish that can be cooked quickly but is tender will be suitable. Examples include:
- pork fillet, butterfly pork steaks, lean pork chops
- beef rump, fillet, stir fry strips
- skinless chicken breast or thighs
- kangaroo fillets or steaks
- fish—any firm-fleshed fish—flathead tails, flake, blue grenadier are just examples
- seafood—seafood mix, calamari, prawns, crab.

Step 3: Add plenty of vegetables

Allow 1½ cups raw per person

Vegetables need to be cut so they are of reasonably even size—strips and angle cuts are good. Fork-sized or bite-sized pieces are best.

Vegetables that take a little extra cooking may be par-cooked first (here's where the microwave oven is so useful): carrots, cauliflower and broccoli fall into this group. Make sure you only just par cook them so they don't finish up soggy and a poor colour.

Try any combination of the following vegetables included in the list below:
- broccoli florets or broccolini
- bean shoots, bamboo shoots, water chestnuts
- beans
- bok choy
- cabbage, Chinese cabbage, shredded
- capsicum, green or red, cut into strips
- carrots, cut into thin strips or rings
- cauliflower florets
- celery
- mushrooms

- onions—spring, Spanish, brown, cut larger onions into rings or chunks
- snow peas, sugar snap peas.

Stir-frying is also a great way to use up vegetables from the 'bottom of the fridge'—that you might otherwise make into soup or even throw away.

> **Time saver**
>
> In a hurry? Try the assorted mixtures of vegetables from the freezer in your supermarket— great if you are cooking for 1 or 2 people.
>
> Check the supermarket shelves or specialty grocers for minces or pastes of chilli, garlic, ginger and shallots. There are also plenty of curry pastes, and packets, cans or jars of spices, pastes and sauces that offer a variety of different flavours. Check the food label and choose low-fat products.

Step 4: Choose your flavours

Try combinations of your own by tasting as you go—if it tastes good before you add it to the stir fry, it will taste good when cooked! You can also buy pre-mixed stir fry sauces but make sure they aren't high in fat or sugar. All are high in salt so use sparingly. Check out the following list for flavour:

- chilli (chopped, minced, fresh or dry)
- coriander—chopped fresh
- 5-spice powder
- garlic—chopped, minced, powder
- ginger—freshly grated, minced
- hoi sin sauce
- lemon grass, finely sliced
- lemon or lime juice
- oyster sauce
- plum sauce
- soy sauce—use a light one to reduce salt intake
- sugar or honey
- sweet chilli sauce
- teriyaki sauce or marinade.

These can either be used to marinate the meat or fish (this adds flavour and helps tenderise the meat), or can be added towards the end of cooking time. Marinades can also be added to the stir fry—just make sure they have boiled before serving the dish.

Flavour

You can increase or decrease the flavour intensity of recipes to suit your own taste. Experiment with herbs and spices; cut back or add more as you like. Such flavour-enhancers will not alter the nutritional value of your food.

If the stir-fry mixture looks a little 'wet' it may need to be thickened. In this case mix 2–3 teaspoons cornflour (cornstarch), potato flour, or arrowroot to a smooth paste with 2 tablespoons cold water. Remove stir-fry from heat, add the well blended thickener and water mixture, then return to the heat and quickly stir over high heat until the mixture thickens. Serve immediately

Step 5: Consider the fat

A small amount of oil is used to cook a stir-fry: 1 tablespoon for 4 people should be plenty. Stir frying uses high heat, so use an oil that has a high flash point—rice bran oil, peanut oil and sesame oil are all good, or even canola. Olive oil is not the best choice for this style of cooking.

Salt

Follow the good health guideline of 'choose foods low in salt'. However, we use common sense, and where we feel that a recipe needs a little salt we add it or use low-salt soy sauce or stock cubes. We encourage you to minimise or omit salt wherever possible. Where we refer to soy sauce in the recipes, we suggest you use 'light' or salt-reduced soy sauce when cooking stir-fries.

The vegetables in stir-fries should be crisp and brightly coloured—the result of swift cooking over high heat. You can substitute other vegetables for the ones listed in the following recipes—this is a good way to use up vegetables. Following are four stir-fry recipes to get you started.

Seafood stir-fry

Serves 4
Preparation/cooking time:
25 minutes

500g (1lb) mixed seafood

2 red chillies, de-seeded and
finely chopped, or 1 teaspoon
minced chilli

1 teaspoon finely chopped
or minced fresh ginger

1 tablespoon light soy sauce

1 teaspoon sugar

200g (7oz) thin spaghetti
or noodles

1 onion, peeled and sliced

½ cup sliced Chinese
or green cabbage

1 cup snow peas or green beans,
topped and tailed

1 red capsicum, seeded and sliced

½ cup thinly sliced mushrooms

½ cup bean sprouts

2 teaspoons sesame oil if
available, otherwise any oil will do

½ cup water

2 teaspoons cornflour

2 tablespoons water

Salt (optional) and ground black
pepper to taste

Method

1. Combine seafood with chilli, ginger, sugar and soy sauce, marinate for ten minutes. Drain juices and reserve.
2. Cook spaghetti or noodles until tender, drain, rinse and keep warm.
3. While pasta is cooking, combine all vegetables except bean sprouts.
4. Heat oil in a wok and lightly stir-fry seafood for about two minutes. Remove from wok and keep warm.
5. Place stock and reserved juices in wok, add vegetables, toss, cover, and simmer for about two minutes or until vegetables are just tender and bright in colour. Check flavour, add pepper and/or salt if needed.
6. Combine cornflour and water and mix to form a thin paste, add to vegetables and stir until sauce cooks and thickens.
7. Add drained spaghetti or noodles and seafood to vegetables, stir-fry until warmed through and serve.

Variation: Replace all or part of the mixed seafood with thin strips of pork or chicken, green prawns or tofu. A few almonds or cashew nuts could be added for variety of taste and texture.

Nutrition data per serve:
1578 kJ (377 cal), carbohydrate 47g, protein 33g, fat 5g, saturated fat 1.0g, fibre 5g, sodium 441mg
GI rating: low

Stir-fry pork or chicken

Serves 4
Preparation/cooking time:
30 minutes

500g (1lb) lean pork or skinless
chicken fillets or thighs

1 tablespoon oil

½–1 teaspoon grated ginger

1 clove garlic, crushed or
½ teaspoon minced garlic

Pinch Chinese five spice powder

1 cup small broccoli florets

1 cup small cauliflower florets

½ green capsicum, diced

2 medium carrots, cut into
matchstick shaped pieces

3 spring onions, trimmed
and sliced

20 snow peas

16 button mushrooms, sliced

2 stalks celery, diagonally sliced

1 tablespoon soy sauce

1 tablespoon honey

1 tablespoon tomato sauce

1 tablespoon cornflour
(cornstarch)

½ cup chicken stock

Method

1. Prepare meat by slicing thinly at an angle.
2. In a bowl, combine soy sauce, honey, tomato sauce, cornflour and chicken stock.
3. Heat oil in pan until very hot. Add meat, ginger, garlic and five spice. Stir-fry for three to five minutes. Remove from pan and set aside.
4. Add broccoli, cauliflower, capsicum and carrots to pan. Stir-fry for one to two minutes, making sure that nothing is allowed to over-cook and become limp.
5. Now add the rest of the vegetables and continue stir-frying over high heat for another one to two minutes.
6. Add the meat to the mixture.
7. Add the sauce, bring to the boil, cover, turn down the heat and simmer for two to three minutes only. Stir to prevent the thickening becoming lumpy.
8. Serve on a bed of basmati rice or rice noodles.

Nutrition data per serve:
1118 kJ (267 cal), carbohydrate 15g, protein 32g, fat 8g, saturated fat 1.7g, fibre 5g, sodium 347mg
GI rating: low–med

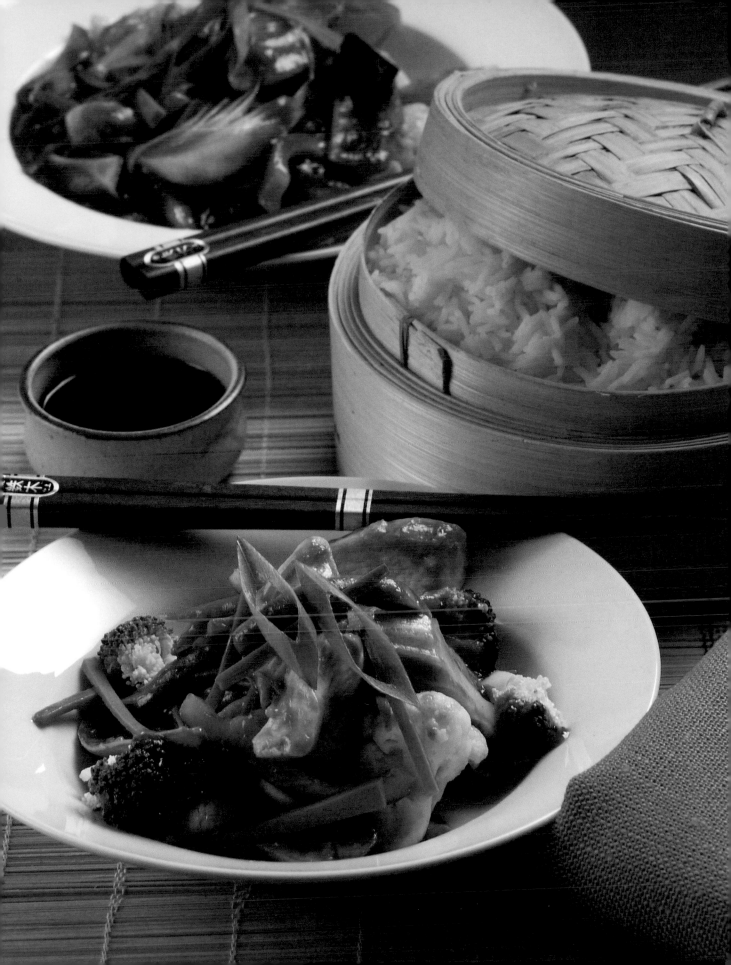

Sweet and sour pork or chicken stir-fry

Serves 4
Preparation/cooking time:
20 minutes

500g (1lb) lean pork or chicken fillets or thighs

2 teaspoons sesame oil if available, otherwise any oil will do

1 bunch spring onions, trimmed and cut into lengths

1 bunch baby bok choy, washed and roughly chopped

1 red capsicum, sliced

2 stalks celery, cut into slices

200g (6½oz) snow peas, trimmed

Sauce:
1 quantity Sweet and sour sauce (recipe page 217)

Method

1. Trim the meat and cut into small chunks.
2. Prepare the vegetables.
3. Heat the oil in a frying pan, add the meat and cook on high heat, stirring often, until browned and cooked through, then set aside.
4. In the same pan cook the onion, bok choy capsicum, celery, and snow peas lightly—the colours should be bright and the vegetables still crunchy, then return the meat to the pan and stir so all ingredients are well mixed.
5. Add the sauce to the meat and vegetables, then return the pan to the heat and stir until warmed and all ingredients thoroughly mixed.
6. Serve with lower GI rice.

Nutrition data per serve: Pork
1523 kJ (364 cal), carbohydrate 21g, protein 25g, fat 19g, saturated fat 6.6g, fibre 4g, sodium 250mg
GI rating: low

Nutrition data per serve: Chicken
1236 kJ (296 cal), carbohydrate 21g, protein 29g, fat 9g, saturated fat 2.5g, fibre 4g, sodium 246mg
GI rating: low

Stir-fry steak
with **black bean** sauce

None of the ingredients in this recipe should be cooked for more than a few minutes.
At the table, the vegetables should still be crisp and retain their true vibrant colour.
Black bean sauce gives a great flavour to this stir fry but is high in sodium.

Serves 4
Preparation/cooking time:
30 minutes

2 teaspoons oil

500g (1lb) beef fillet or lean rump
steak, trimmed of fat
or 500g (1lb) stir-fry beef strips

1 medium onion, peeled
and quartered

¼ cup coarsely chopped green
capsicum

¼ cup coarsely chopped red
capsicum

1 medium carrot, sliced

½ cup commercial black
bean sauce

Method

1. Brush oil over the base of a frying pan or wok and heat over high heat.
2. Slice steak into very thin strips, about 3–4 centimetres (1½ inches) long and ½ centimetres (¼ inch) wide.
3. Sauté quickly for about 3 minutes.
4. Add vegetables and stir-fry for a further two minutes.
5. Add black bean sauce, cover and simmer gently for 5 minutes.
6. Serve with boiled rice.

Nutrition data per serve:
1031 kJ (246 cal), carbohydrate 11g, protein 28g, fat 9g, saturated fat 3.2g, fibre 2g, sodium 1413mg
GI rating: low

Other stir-fry recipes can be found in other sections of this book, e.g.: Stir-fried Bok Choy with Fish and Almonds page 129.

Balanced eating: carbohydrate

Carbohydrate foods should form an important part of your eating pattern as the sugars and starches in foods maintain the blood glucose levels and provide much of the energy that your body needs.

Recipes high in carbohydrate have been grouped together according to the major carbohydrate food the dish contains:

- rice
- pasta and noodles
- pancakes

- potato
- couscous, polenta, gnocchi and cracked wheat
- starchy vegetables.

Rice dishes

Where possible, choose lower GI rice (see pages 23 and 277).

Basic risotto

First we give you a basic risotto and then show you how to make it more interesting.

Serves 4
Preparation/cooking time:
30–40 minutes

1 tablespoon margarine

1 teaspoon minced garlic

2 onions, peeled and finely chopped

1¼ cups arborio rice

4-5 cups Basic homemade chicken stock (page 89) and 1 cup dry white wine

Pepper and salt to taste (optional)

2 tablespoons parsley, chopped

2 tablespoons parmesan cheese, grated, for garnish

Method

1. Heat stock and keep hot while the risotto is being prepared.
2. Melt margarine in a large saucepan on medium heat.
3. Add the garlic and onion, and cook until translucent—stir enough to avoid sticking and burning—this takes 2–3 minutes.
4. Add the rice and stir again until the rice grains start to whiten.
5. Add 1 cup hot stock, stir occasionally while the rice absorbs the stock. At this point, add the meat if using.
6. When the mixture thickens, add a further cup of stock and allow to absorb into the rice.
7. Add the first of the vegetables and stir in—this will be the vegetables that take a little longer to cook such as pumpkin, sweet potato, carrot, mushroom, sweetcorn, sun-dried tomatoes, broccoli florets (it is preferable to at least par-cook these (except tomatoes) to make sure they are cooked through by the time the risotto is ready to serve).

Plus: vegetables, meat or fish and flavour ingredients of your choice— use the ideas below (with suggested amounts) to get you started.

8. Add another cup of stock and stir often enough to prevent sticking/burning—this will absorb as before.
9. At this point, add the final vegetables such as beans, snow peas, spinach, asparagus, peas, and any fresh herbs like basil, parsley, chives.
10. Add the last of the stock and the salt and pepper and allow the stock to absorb into the rice—the rice mixture should be creamy, with a little 'sauce' at this point—not stiff and dry. If so, add some extra stock or vegetable juice (liquid from cooking vegetables, corn liquor etc), then serve, with extra parsley if you wish, topped with parmesan cheese.

Vegetables: any combinations work really well with a risotto. You can even use frozen mixed vegetables or leftover roast vegetables. Allow 2 cups vegetables for 4 serves.

If using meat or fish: reduce vegetables to 2–3 cups for 4 serves. Prior to sautéing the onion and garlic at step 3, sauté or par cook the meat or fish in a little of the margarine. Set aside. Add the meat with the first cup of stock at step 5 to ensure it has time to cook. The seafood should be almost cooked during sautéing and so is best added with the vegetables at step 9.

Risotto will freeze, but you may need to add extra stock or water when you re-heat it, as it will have thickened on standing.

The addition of vegetables to this basic risotto will increase the fibre content of this recipe. For instance, 2 cups of frozen green peas and corn adds 5g fibre per serve.

Nutrition data per serve:
1193 kJ (285 cal), carbohydrate 52g, protein 6g, fat 5g, saturated fat 1.3g, fibre 1g, sodium 81mg
GI rating: med

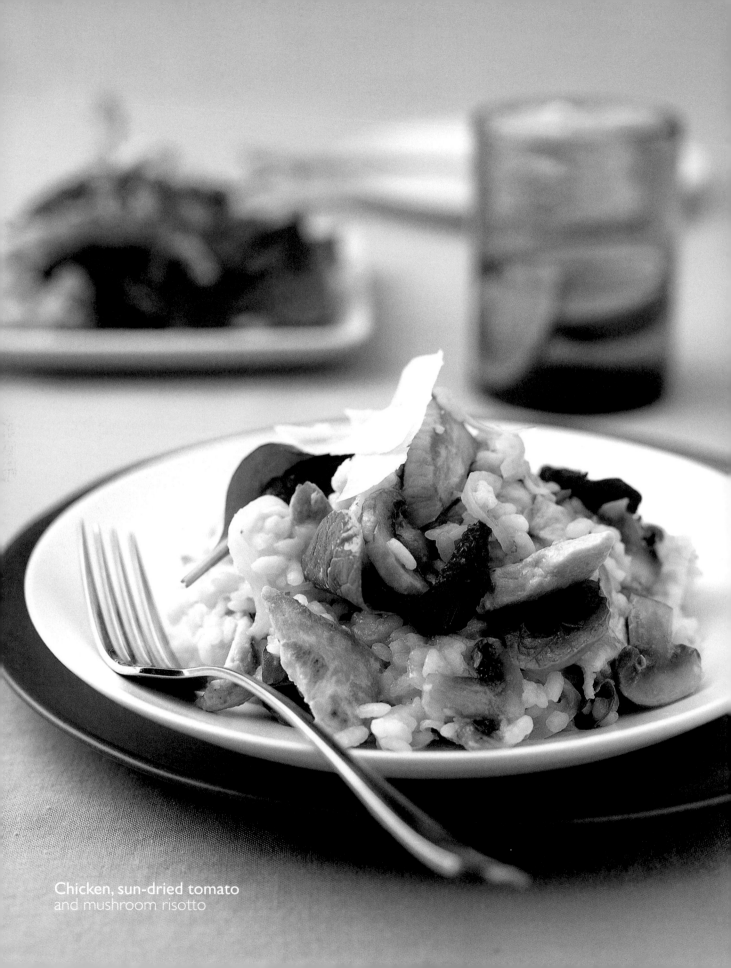

Chicken, sun-dried tomato
and mushroom risotto

Chicken, sun-dried tomato
and mushroom risotto

Serves 4
Preparation/cooking time:
40 minutes

To the basic risotto add:

2 chicken fillets, cut into bite-size
pieces

½ cup semi-dried tomatoes,
cut in half

1 cup button mushrooms

Black pepper, to taste

4 cups baby spinach leaves

2 rounded tablespoons low-fat
ricotta cheese

Method

1. Sauté the chicken in a little of the margarine and set aside.
   Add at Step 5 as per Basic Risotto.
2. Follow the basic risotto method as above, adding tomatoes
   and mushrooms at Step 7 and spinach at Step 9.
3. Fold the ricotta cheese in as you are ready to serve.

Nutrition data per serve:
1943 kJ (463 cal), carbohydrate 60g, protein 27g, fat 11g, saturated
fat 3.4g, fibre 5g, sodium 170mg
GI rating: med

Seafood risotto

Serves 4
Preparation/cooking time:
40 minutes

To the basic risotto add:

2 cups mixed seafood (white fish,
prawns, scallops, mussels, crab
meat and/or oysters)

1 cup button mushrooms

1 cup green beans, sliced

1 bunch bok choy, washed and
roughly chopped

2 rounded tablespoons ricotta
cheese

Method

1. Sauté the seafood in a little of the margarine and set aside.
2. Follow the Basic Risotto method, add seafood, mushrooms,
   green beans and bok choy at Step 9.
3. Fold in the ricotta cheese and sprinkle with parsley as you
   are ready to serve.

Nutrition data per serve:
1649 kJ (394 cal), carbohydrate 59g, protein 20g, fat 7g, saturated
fat 2.1g, fibre 5g, sodium 322mg
GI rating: med

Fried rice

This recipe works well as an accompaniment to meat dishes, or as a light meal/lunch dish on its own.

Serves 6
Preparation/cooking time:
30 minutes

1½ cups Mahatma™ white long grain or other lower GI rice

2 eggs

2 tablespoons water

Pepper and salt to taste (optional)

2 teaspoons oil—preferably sesame or peanut oil if available

1 teaspoon 5-spice powder or 1 teaspoon curry powder

1 cup celery, chopped finely

12 spring onions, trimmed and sliced finely

1 red capsicum, chopped finely

1 green capsicum, chopped finely

1 cup frozen peas

1 small carrot, grated

½ cup snow peas or beans, trimmed and sliced into short lengths

1 cup frozen sweetcorn kernels

2 slices lean ham, chopped into small pieces

3–4 teaspoons low-salt ('lite') soy sauce

2 teaspoons sweet chilli sauce (optional)

Method

1. Cook rice, drain and rinse to remove excess starch, set aside.
2. While rice is cooking, prepare the vegetables and set aside.
3. Beat the eggs with 2 tablespoons water, add pepper and salt to taste.
4. Cook the eggs in a frying pan sprayed with a little oil.
5. When set, remove from heat and slice into strips.
6. Place sesame oil in a large frying pan or Wok and heat, add 5-spice powder and cook a few seconds, stirring, to release the aromas. Add the vegetables, return to the heat, and cook, stirring, until the vegetables are cooked but still crunchy.
7. Add the rice, egg and ham, stir again to combine flavours, add the soy sauce (and sweet chilli sauce if using), check flavour and adjust as needed.
8. Serve hot.

Nutrition data per serve:
1154 kJ (276 cal), carbohydrate 46g, protein 10g, fat 4g, saturated fat 1g, fibre 5g, sodium 284mg
GI rating: low

Spiced rice with peas

This dish is a colourful and tasty accompaniment to any spicy meat dish—particularly curries
—try serving it with Indian lamb in spinach sauce (page 196)

Serves 4
Preparation/cooking time:
25 minutes

1 tablespoon vegetable oil

1 teaspoon finely chopped fresh
ginger or minced ginger

½ fresh chilli, finely chopped,
or ½ teaspoon minced chilli paste

¼ teaspoon black mustard seeds

¼ teaspoon cumin seeds

3 cups water

2 curry leaves (optional)

1 cup Mahatma™ white long grain
or basmati rice

2 cups frozen peas

1½ tablespoons of one or
combination of fresh coriander,
mint, and basil, chopped

¼ teaspoon ground saffron
(optional)

Salt to taste (optional)

Method

1. Heat oil in pan, add ginger, chilli, mustard and cumin seeds
   and cook, stirring, for one minute.
2. Add water, bring to boil and add all other ingredients, cover
   and return to boil.
3. Reduce heat and simmer for 15 minutes or until rice is tender.

See photo on page 152.

Nutrition data per serve:
1145 kJ (274 cal), carbohydrate 46g, protein 8g, fat 5g, saturated
fat 0.6g, fibre 5g, sodium 5mg
GI rating: low

Rice desserts can provide useful carbohydrate if a meal is low in carbohydrate
Although rice is mainly used in savoury dishes it makes an easy and popular dessert which
can be particularly useful if the main course of the meal does not provide an adequate
amount of carbohydrate, (see pages 225 and 230).

Pasta dishes and sauces

Pasta is low in GI

Most pasta is made from wheat with a high protein content (known as hard wheat) which forms a dense product and slows digestion and absorption. This makes most pasta low in GI value and a good choice for people with diabetes. If eating pasta away from home, take care as many dishes are served only with a little sauce and few accompaniments and the size of the pasta serving is often large.

In our recipes we have allowed 80 grams (3 ounces) of raw pasta per serve.

Pasta comes in all shapes and sizes from the large, flat rectangular pasta of lasagne, to the long tubes of traditional spaghetti, the fine strands of angel hair, the short thick tubes of cannelloni and the small tubes of macaroni to the flat ribbons of fettuccine, tagliatelle or linguini. Other varieties include shapes like twists, spirals, butterflies, bowties, snails, shells, small rings and stuffed pastas like tortellini and ravioli. Try different varieties. If your sauce has a delicate flavour, a thin pasta may be best; or if you are trying to trap the sauce and all its flavour the ones with twists may be better.

Pasta sauces

The sauces we give you here are adaptable—try them with pasta or noodles, gnocchi, or in pancakes or over jacket potatoes. Serve with salad and grainy bread.

Creamy corn sauce

This recipe is quick and easy to make, and blends well with a variety of pasta types.

Serves 4
Preparation/cooking time:
20 minutes

2 teaspoons margarine

6 spring onions, trimmed and chopped into small rings

400g (14oz) can creamed corn

¾ cup low-fat evaporated milk

2 tablespoons chopped parsley or chives or basil or coriander

Salt (optional) and pepper to taste

1 tablespoon cornflour (cornstarch)

3 tablespoons water

Method

1. Melt margarine in a saucepan, add the spring onions and cook for 1–2 minutes, stirring to prevent burning.
2. Add the corn, the evaporated milk, stock powder, pepper and salt to taste, and the fresh herbs. Bring to boil then turn heat down and allow to simmer for a few minutes. Remove from heat.
3. Combine the cornstarch with water, blend until smooth, then add to the corn mixture, mixing in well.
4. Return sauce to the heat and bring to the boil again, then simmer, stirring to prevent lumps forming, until the sauce has thickened.

Nutrition data per serve:
700 kJ (167 cal), carbohydrate 25g, protein 6g, fat 4g, saturated fat 1g, fibre 4g, sodium 375mg
GI rating: med

Bolognese sauce

This sauce works well with a variety of pasta dishes—it not only makes a tasty spaghetti bolognese, but can be used to fill instant cannelloni tubes or as the filling for lasagne, or simply adapted to make a filling for tacos or burritos, a topping for jacket potatoes, or a meat pie filling. It freezes well.

Serves 4
Preparation/cooking time:
45 minutes

2 teaspoons oil, preferably extra virgin olive

2 large onions, peeled and chopped finely

4 cloves garlic, crushed, or 2 teaspoons minced garlic

500g (1lb) lean minced beef

4 tablespoons tomato paste

1 x 400g (14oz) can peeled or crushed tomatoes

½ cup red wine (optional) +1 cup water or 1½ cups water

2 teaspoons Italian or mixed dried herbs

2 teaspoons sugar (this balances the acidity of tomatoes)

Salt and pepper to taste (optional)

Method
1. Heat oil in a deep frying pan.
2. Add onion and garlic, cook until slightly browned.
3. Add the meat, stir to break up any lumps while it browns.
4. Add the tomato paste, the tomatoes, the stock powder, water and/or wine, the herbs, sugar, and salt and pepper to taste. Stir until all ingredients are well mixed—break up any lumps of tomato or meat. Reduce heat and simmer, covered, until the sauce is cooked and fairly smooth—the cooking time is needed to blend the flavours and develop richness of flavour.

Note: the final sauce should be reasonably runny for spaghetti sauce or as a filling for lasagne.

If you plan to use the sauce for cannelloni filling, filling for burritos or tacos, or as chilli con carne, allow it to cook longer with the lid off to thicken by evaporation.

Nutrition data per serve:
1147 kJ (274 cal), carbohydrate 12g, protein 29g, fat 11g, saturated fat 4g, fibre 4g, sodium 309mg
GI rating: low

The Bolognese sauce can be varied for tacos or burritos:
1. Leave out the wine and use 1½ cups water.
2. Add one 300g (10 ½oz) tomato-based salsa or ½ packet of taco seasoning mix at Step 4 (according to taste). This slightly thickens the sauce as well as adding spiciness.

For Chilli con carne: Add 400g (14oz) red kidney beans, drained and rinsed to above and top with chopped onions.

Fresh tomato sauce

Serves 4
Preparation/cooking time:
20 minutes

2 teaspoons olive oil

1 medium onion, finely chopped

2 cloves garlic, crushed,
or 2 teaspoons minced garlic

500g (1lb) ripe tomatoes, chopped

2 tablespoons tomato paste

½ teaspoon dried oregano
or Italian herbs

Ground black pepper

½ cup water

½ cup dry white wine

2 tablespoons chopped fresh basil

Method

1. Heat oil in saucepan, add onion and garlic and sauté until translucent.
2. Add tomatoes, tomato paste, water, wine, dried herbs and pepper and simmer for ten to fifteen minutes, or until the sauce is fairly thick and the tomatoes well broken down.
3. Add the fresh basil and serve.

Nutrition data per total quantity:
323 kJ (77 cal), carbohydrate 5g, protein 2g, fat 2g, saturated fat 0.3g, fibre 2g, sodium 88mg
GI rating: low

Spinach and ricotta sauce or filling

This mixture is very versatile. You can fold it through pasta, but it works very well as a filling for cannelloni or lasagne, or used to make spinach triangles or spinach pie.

Serves 4
Preparation/cooking time:
20 minutes

1 bunch fresh spinach
or 1 x 250g (8¾oz) package
frozen spinach

450g (16oz) fresh low-fat ricotta
cheese

8 spring onions, trimmed and
chopped finely

1 teaspoon mixed dried herbs
or oregano

½–1 teaspoon ground nutmeg

1 teaspoon garlic (optional)

1 egg, beaten

4 tablespoons freshly grated
Parmesan cheese

2 tablespoons fresh basil, chopped
(omit when making this mixture
for spinach triangles)

Method

1. Thaw and drain the frozen spinach. If using fresh, trim off the stalks and place leaves in a saucepan.
2. Wilt over medium heat (lid on), then cool, drain, and chop.
3. Add the ricotta cheese to a mixing bowl, crumble well.
4. Add the spinach, onions, herbs and spice, garlic if using, the egg, and the parmesan cheese, mix all together well. Check flavour and add pepper to taste.

Storage: this will keep for up to 2 days covered in the refrigerator if not using immediately. It will freeze as part of a cooked dish.

Note: if making spinach pie (see page 165), use this recipe but increase frozen spinach to 2 x 250g (8¾oz) packages, or use 2 bunches spinach if using fresh spinach.

Nutrition data per serve:
947 kJ (226 cal), carbohydrate 5g, protein 20g, fat 14g, saturated fat 8.1g, fibre 4g, sodium 354mg
GI rating: low

Tomato and chickpea sauce

The currants and Eastern spices seem an odd combination for a pasta sauce, but the flavours go very well together and the currants provide a piquant touch that really adds to the final flavour of the sauce—try it!

Serves 4
Preparation/cooking time:
40 minutes

2 teaspoons olive oil

1 teaspoon minced garlic

2 medium onions, peeled and finely chopped

1/8 teaspoon ground cloves

1 teaspoon ground cumin

1 teaspoon ground coriander

1 teaspoon ground garam masala

400g (14oz) can chickpeas, drained and rinsed

440g (15fl oz) can no-added-salt tomatoes in tomato juice, chopped

4 tablespoons no-salt tomato paste

½ cup currants

2 tablespoons chopped fresh parsley

Method

1. Heat oil in large saucepan, add the spices, garlic and onions and cook, stirring, until the onions are soft.
2. Add the chickpeas, currants, pasta sauce, tomato paste and parsley and simmer on low heat with the lid on for 30 minutes to allow the flavours to develop and blend.
3. Serve as a sauce with pasta, or use as a filling for lasagne (see page 142).

Nutrition data per serve:
943 kJ (226 cal), carbohydrate 35g, protein 9g, fat 3g, saturated fat 0.5g, fibre 10g, sodium 366mg
GI rating: low

Vegetarian lasagne

Serves 6
Preparation/cooking time:
60 minutes

200g (7oz) instant lasagne sheets

1 x 810g (29oz) can no-added-salt tomatoes in tomato juice, chopped

4 tablespoons no-added-salt tomato paste

½ quantity tomato and chickpea sauce

½ quantity spinach and ricotta filling

1 cup low-fat mozzarella cheese, grated

Method

1. Preheat oven to 180°C (350°F)
2. Combine tomatoes and tomato paste.
3. Spread ½ the tomato mixture over the base of a square or rectangular casserole dish.
4. Place lasagne sheets over the sauce.
5. Spread the tomato and chickpea sauce over the sheets.
6. Cover with another layer of pasta sheets.
7. Spread the ricotta and spinach mixture over the pasta sheets.
8. Cover with a final layer of pasta sheets.
9. Spread the remaining ½ of the tomato mixture over the top, making sure you cover the pasta sheets.
10. Sprinkle with the mozzarella cheese.
11. Bake until the top is lightly browned and the pasta seems tender if pierced with a sharp knife.

Variation: replace the top layer of pasta sauce with a white sauce (see page 215), and top with 2 tablespoons grated Parmesan cheese.

Nutrition data per serve:
1529 kJ (366cal), carbohydrate 44g, protein 21g, fat 10g, saturated fat 5g, fibre 9g, sodium 391mg
GI rating: low

Salads containing pasta can be found in Lunches and light meals (see page 88)

Spinach and ricotta cannelloni

This recipe uses ½ the quantity of Spinach and ricotta filling. If you make the full quantity of filling, the other half can be used as 1 layer in a lasagne, or to make spinach triangles (see page 259)

Serves 4
Preparation/cooking time:
20 minutes for filling,
10 minutes to fill cannelloni,
30–40 minutes cooking time

12 instant cannelloni tubes

1 x 810g can no added salt tomatoes in tomato juice, chopped

4 tablespoons no-added-salt tomato paste

½ quantity spinach and ricotta filling (page 140)

1 cup low-fat mozzarella cheese, grated (optional)

2 tablespoons parsley, chopped

Method

1. Preheat oven to 180ºC (350ºF)
2. Combine tomatoes and tomato paste.
3. Place ½ the tomato mixture over the base of a square or rectangular casserole dish.
4. Fill the cannelloni tubes with spinach and ricotta mixture, place in the dish.
5. Pour the remainder of the tomato mixture over the top, spreading evenly.
6. If using the mozzarella cheese, sprinkle over the top.
7. Bake until the top is lightly browned and the pasta is tender if pierced with a sharp knife.
8. Remove from the oven and garnish with chopped parsley.

Nutrition data per serve:
1468 kJ, (350 cal), carbohydrate 45g, protein 19g, fat 10g, saturated fat 5.0g, fibre 7g, sodium 1174mg
GI rating: low

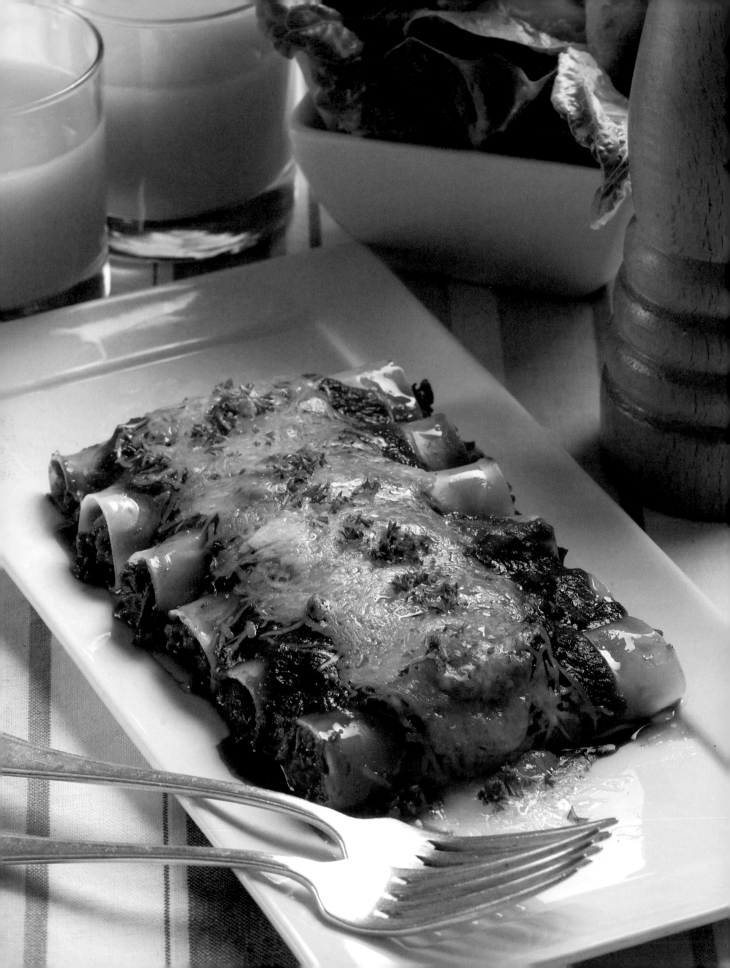

Meat cannelloni

Serves 4
Preparation/cooking time:
50 minutes + sauce
preparation

12 instant cannelloni tubes

1 x 810g (29oz) can no-added-salt
tomatoes in tomato
juice, chopped

4 tablespoons no-added-salt
tomato paste

½ quantity bolognese sauce
(see comments page 138
sauce needs to be thick)

1 cup low fat mozzarella
cheese, grated

2 tablespoons parmesan cheese

2 tablespoons chopped fresh
parsley

Method

1. Preheat oven to 180°C (350°F)
2. Combine tomatoes and tomato paste
3. Spread ½ tomato mixture over the base of a square or rectangular casserole dish.
4. Fill each tube with meat mixture, place on the tomato mixture.
5. Spread the rest of the tomato mixture over the tubes, sprinkle with mozzarella and Parmesan, and bake until the top is lightly browned and the pasta seems tender when pierced with a sharp knife—30–40 minutes average cooking time.
6. Serve sprinkled with chopped parsley.

Nutrition data per serve:
1665 kJ (398 cal), carbohydrate 41g, protein 29g, fat 12g, saturated fat 5.6g, fibre 7g, sodium 384mg
GI rating: low

Potato dishes

Potatoes form an important part of many peoples' eating patterns and are a good source of carbohydrate. Potatoes have high GI rating so choose small servings. Try to include at least one food with a low GI in the same meal as potatoes as this will lower the GI rating of the meal.

Dry curry of potato, eggplant and pea

Serves 4
Preparation/cooking time:
45 minutes

1 tablespoon margarine

1½ teaspoons panch phora (Indian five spices)—optional

1 large onion, finely chopped

2 tablespoons chopped mint

1 teaspoon finely chopped fresh ginger

¼ teaspoon ground chilli

1 teaspoon ground turmeric

500g (1lb) potatoes, peeled and diced

500g (1lb) eggplant (aubergine), diced

250g (8¾oz) frozen or fresh green peas

3 tablespoons hot water

1 teaspoon garam masala

1 tablespoon lemon juice

Salt to taste (optional)

Method

1. Heat the margarine and fry the panch phora until seeds start to brown.
2. Add onion and fry until soft.
3. Add mint, ginger, chilli and turmeric and stir.
4. Add vegetables and water, mix well and cover.
5. Reduce to a low heat and cook for 20 minutes, shaking pan occasionally to toss vegetables and to prevent them burning.
6. Sprinkle with garam masala, lemon juice and salt, cover and cook for a further 10 minutes.
7. Serve hot.

Panch phora is a mixture of 5 different seeds used whole—one part each of fenu greek seeds and fennel seeds, two parts each of black mustard seeds, cumin seeds and black cumin seeds. Garam Masala is a mixture of ground spices such as coriander, cumin, cardamom, cinnamon, cloves and nutmeg. Both blends can be purchased pre-mixed.

Nutrition data per serve:
871 kJ (208 cal), carbohydrate 29g, protein 9g, fat 4g, saturated fat 0.6g, fibre 9g, sodium 37mg
GI rating: high

Potato Gnocchi

Any type of potato can be used in this recipe although Nicola or an alternative waxy potato is best.

Serves 4 (10 pieces per serve)
Preparation/cooking time:
20 minutes

750g (1¾lb) potatoes

1 cup plain flour

2 eggs, lightly beaten

1 quantity of Fresh tomato sauce
(see page 139)

Method

1. Peel and cook potatoes by simmering in water until soft. Cooking water may be lightly salted if desired. Drain.

2. Half fill saucepan with fresh water and place on stove to boil. A little salt may be added to the cooking water if desired.

3. Once potatoes are cool enough to handle, press through a potato ricer or mouli or mash with a potato masher.

4. Spread ¾ cup flour onto bench top or large board and top with potato.

5. Add eggs and quickly mix all ingredients together to form a light, smooth dough.

6. Divide mixture into four, turn onto a clean bench top or large board which has been sprinkled with remaining flour and roll each into a sausage shape about 2 centimetres (¾ inch) in diameter. Cut lengths into 2-centimetre pieces and press each top lightly with a fork.

7. Drop gnocchi pieces into boiling water in small batches. Allow to boil, without lid, until they float to the surface (about ½–1 min).

8. Use a slotted spoon to remove onto a serving dish and top with fresh tomato sauce.

Nutrition data per serve:
1455 kJ (348 cal), carbohydrate 52g, protein 13g, fat 6g, saturated fat 1.2g, fibre 6g, sodium 127mg
GI rating: high

......and the sauce

Potato gnocchi has a high GI. This is a good example of how the accompanying food, in this case the sauce, can be used to lower the GI of the dish. The acid in a tomato based sauce, such as Fresh tomato page 139, milk in a milk based sauce, such as Cheese sauce page 216, or a meat-based sauce which provides some fat, such as Bolognese sauce page 138, will all help to slow the digestion and absorption of the starch in the potato.

Pancakes

An under-used but quick and delicious meal is pancakes. Here we show you how to make these and suggest some creative fillings using meat, fish or vegetables. These delectable packages can be eaten fresh, or frozen and reheated at a moment's notice.

Thin pancakes or crêpes

Serves 4 (2 per serve)
Makes 8 thin pancakes approx
15cm (6in) in diameter
Preparation/cooking time:
20 minutes + 1 hour standing
time for batter

½ cup plain white flour

½ cup wholemeal flour

1 egg, lightly beaten

1½ cups low-fat or skim milk

1 tablespoon oil for cooking

Method

1. Place flours into a bowl and make a well in the centre.
2. Slowly add the beaten egg and then the milk, stirring continually to draw the ingredients together and prevent lumps forming. Mixture should form a thin, smooth pouring consistency (like pouring cream). If you prefer, use a food processor or blender, add all the ingredients at once and process until smooth.
3. Leave to stand in a cool place for at least an hour. If the mixture has thickened too much, add more milk, a little at a time, to the consistency of thin pouring cream.
4. Lightly grease a heavy bottomed frying pan with 1 teaspoon oil and heat until very hot, but not smoking. Pour in 4 tablespoons of batter and tilt pan to spread batter evenly.
5. When fine bubbles appear on the surface of the pancake and it appears dry, use an egg slice or spatula to flip over and cook the other side for a few seconds until pale golden brown on both sides.
6. Repeat these steps for the remainder of the batter, brushing the pan with ¼–½ teaspoon oil between crêpes and stacking them as they are cooked. Keep them covered with a damp tea-towel until you need them.
7. Use any of the filling mixtures listed below, or create your own. Crêpes and pancakes can be filled and then served rolled up or folded in half or in quarters.

Storage: Cover and refrigerate for up to two days, or pack in freezer bags, with a layer of waxed paper or plastic film between each crêpe, and freeze.

Nutrition data per serve (2 pancakes):
891 kJ (213 cal), carbohydrate 28g, protein 9g, fat 6g, saturated fat 1.2g, fibre 3g, sodium 61mg
GI rating: low

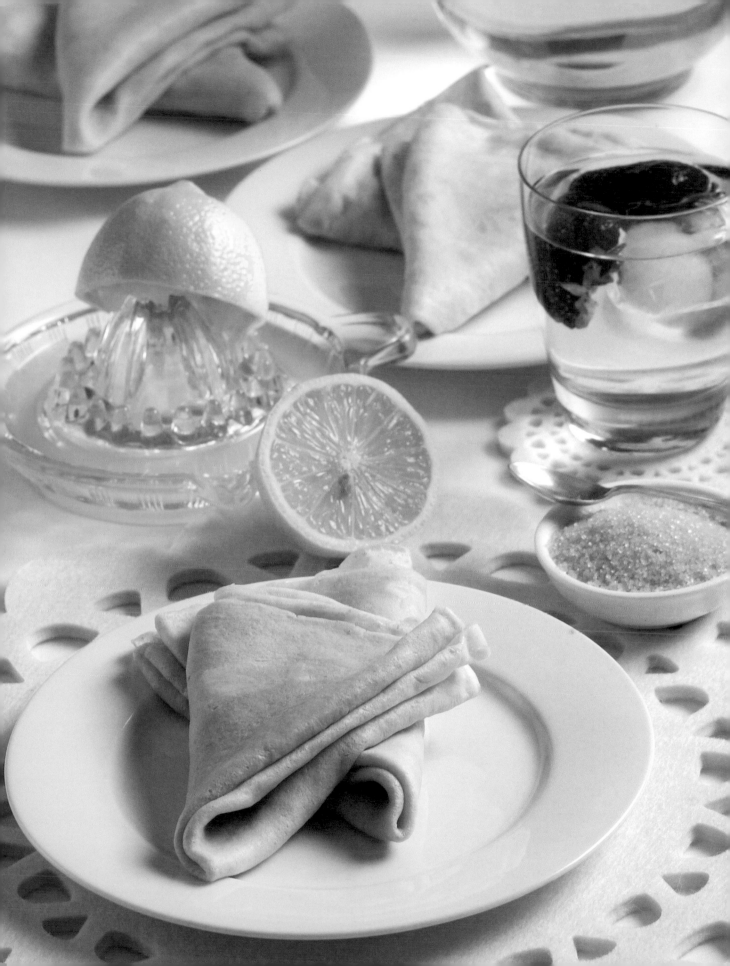

Savoury fillings for thin pancakes or crêpes

Allow two pancakes per serve.

Fill pancakes (see suggestions that follow) and top with low-fat natural yoghurt, low-fat ricotta cheese or a fine sprinkling of parmesan cheese. Serve the filled pancakes hot, accompanied by a crisp, green salad.

Several recipes in this book make great fillings:

- Bolognese sauce—see page 138
- Spinach and ricotta filling—see page 140
- Mushroom stroganoff—see page 110
- Tomato and chickpea sauce—see page 141
- Creamy corn sauce—see page 137
- Beef stroganoff—see page 195

Or create your own fillings, for example:

Mix cooked or canned asparagus spears or cooked chicken fillets and avocado with cheese sauce—see page 216.

Pancakes are also great for breakfasts, lunches, dessert or parties and special occasions. Look for sweet filled or topped pancakes in other sections of this book:

- Breakfast: Apple and sultana pancakes—see page 76
- Desserts and sweet treats: Berry and cheese pancakes—see page 233
- Special occasion meals: Flambéed crepes and Crêpes suzette—see page 271

Starchy vegetables and other carbohydrates

Starchy vegetables, with the exception of regular potato and other carbohydrate-rich foods such as couscous, polenta, semolina and cracked wheat, are medium to low GI. They make great additions to your eating plan especially when served with a tomato, meat or legume sauce which help to lower the GI further.

Sweet potato salad

This 'salad' is just as tasty served hot or cold, and is really versatile—it goes well with a wide variety of main dishes, or you can enjoy it alone as a light meal.

Serves 6
Preparation/cooking time:
20 minutes

2 medium sweet potatoes

300g (10½oz) green beans

200g (7oz) snow peas

12 spring onions or 1 large red onion

2 teaspoons sesame oil

1 teaspoon grated or minced fresh ginger

Dressing:

1 tablespoon sesame oil

4 tablespoons lime juice (lemon if no lime available)

1 tablespoon sweet chilli sauce

1 tablespoon sugar

1 teaspoon freshly grated or minced ginger

2 tablespoons fresh coriander

Method

1. Peel the sweet potato, cut into ½ centimetre (¼ inch) thick slices, and cook until just tender in the microwave. Set aside.
2. Trim the beans and cut into 3–4 centimetre (1–1½ inch) lengths, then cook in the microwave until just cooked—they should still be bright green and crunchy. Set aside.
3. Chop the onions, and trim the snow peas into 2 centimetre (¾ inch) lengths.
4. Heat the oil in a large frying pan or wok, add the onion, snow peas and ginger and cook, tossing often, until just cooked—this takes no more than 3–4 minutes. Add sweet potato and beans.
5. Make the dressing by combining all ingredients—check flavour and adjust if necessary.
6. Pour the dressing over the vegetables, toss and allow to heat through.

This will keep in a covered container for 1–2 days in the refrigerator.

Nutrition data per serve:
619 kJ (148 cal), carbohydrate 22g, protein 5g, fat 4g, saturated fat 0.5g, fibre 5g, sodium 64mg
GI rating: med

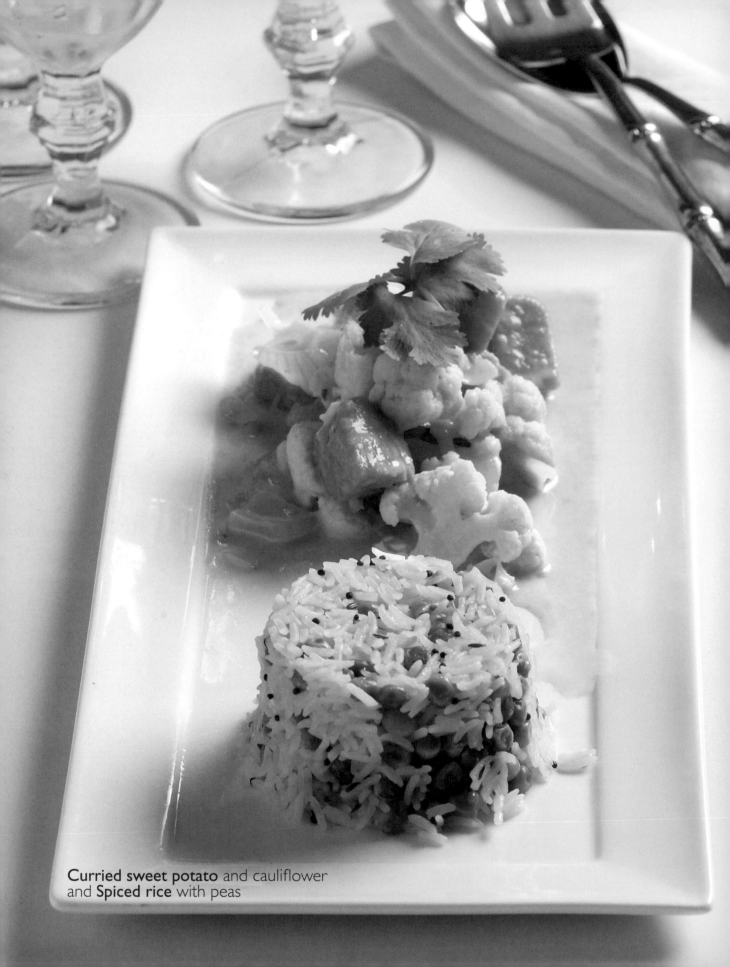

Curried sweet potato and cauliflower
and **Spiced rice** with peas

Curried sweet potato
and cauliflower

The flavour of curried food improves with standing, so this dish can be prepared 24 hours in advance and stored, well covered, in the refrigerator. Reheat before serving.

Serves 4
Preparation/cooking time:
40 minutes

1 moderate–large sweet potato, peeled

½ cauliflower

1 medium onion

2 teaspoons curry powder

1 teaspoon ground cumin

1 teaspoon ground coriander

1 cup light (low-fat) coconut milk

1 teaspoon sugar

Salt to taste (optional)

Chopped parsley or coriander to garnish

Method

1. Cut the vegetables into bite-sized pieces, place in a microwave dish and cook, covered, until just tender.
2. Dry fry the onion and spices for 1–2 minutes. Add the coconut milk and sugar.
3. Add the drained vegetables, mix to combine, then simmer with the lid on 10–15 minutes.
4. Remove the vegetables, placing in a serving dish.
5. Re-heat the liquid, simmering until it has reduced and thickened a little. Check flavour and add a little salt if needed.
6. Serve, garnished with a little chopped parsley or coriander.

Nutrition data per serve:
750 kJ (179 cal), carbohydrate 30g, protein 11g, fat 4g, saturated fat 4.0g, fibre 5g, sodium 101mg
GI rating: med

Succotash

Succotash was originally a Native American dish. This is a quick and easy version.

Serves 4
Preparation/cooking time:
30 minutes

1 cup frozen corn kernels

1 cup frozen peas

1 cup canned or frozen lima beans

1 small red capsicum, chopped

1 quantity White Sauce
(see page 215)

1 tablespoon chopped parsley

Method

1. Cook the peas and corn until just tender, drain.

2. Drain and rinse the lima beans if canned, or cook as for peas and corn, drain.

3. Combine vegetables in a shallow baking dish, pour the sauce over, bake 15 minutes—until the sauce is bubbling, then serve, garnished with chopped parsley.

Nutrition data per serve:
936 kJ (224 cal), carbohydrate 28g, protein 12g, fat 6g, saturated fat 1.6g, fibre 6g, sodium 411mg
GI rating: low

Semolina gnocchi
with mushroom sauce

Gnocchi are best served fresh, but you can refrigerate them for up to three days and then reheat by dropping in boiling water. Alternatively, freeze the uncooked gnocchi and cook when you need to serve them.

Serves 4
Preparation/cooking time:
30 minutes

1½ cups skim or low-fat milk

½ teaspoon ground nutmeg

1 cup semolina

2 eggs

Small amount of plain flour

1 quantity Mushroom stroganoff (see page 110)

Method

1. Place milk and nutmeg in medium saucepan and bring to boil. Remove from heat and quickly stir in semolina.
2. Return to heat and stir for one minute.
3. Add eggs and work into a smooth dough.
4. Break off small, even-sized pieces about the size of a walnut, roll into balls and toss in a little flour.
5. Half fill a large saucepan with water and bring to the boil.
6. Drop gnocchi into boiling water and cook for about five minutes (gnocchi will rise to the top of the water as they cook).
7. Drain. Toss in mushroom sauce and serve immediately.

Storage: Can be refrigerated for up to 3 days and reheated in boiling water. Alternatively, the uncooked gnocchi can be frozen.

Nutrition data per serve:
1247 kJ (298 cal), carbohydrate 43g, protein 19g, fat 4g, saturated fat 1g, fibre 5g, sodium 321mg
GI rating: low

Gnocchi can be made from different ingredients—see Potato gnocchi, page 147

Roast winter
vegetable medley

Serves 4
Preparation/cooking time:
1 hour

1 tablespoons olive oil

1 medium potato, peeled

1 small swede, peeled (optional)

1 small sweet potato, peeled

1 beetroot, peeled

1 parsnip, peeled

1 onion, peeled

Freshly ground black pepper

Salt (optional)

1 tablespoon chopped fresh rosemary

2 teaspoons chopped fresh sage

Method

1. Preheat the oven to 200°C (400°F)
2. Cut each of the vegetables into four pieces and place into a large mixing bowl, add the seasonings and the oil, and toss until the vegetables are well coated with the oil and seasonings.
3. Spread the vegetables over the base of a baking dish, spooning any residual oil over them.
4. Bake until the vegetables are tender and browned, about 45 minutes. Turn the vegetables at least once during the cooking period.

Nutrition data per serve:
698 kJ (167 cal), carbohydrate 24g, protein 4g, fat 5g, saturated fat 0.6g, fibre 6g, sodium 43mg
GI rating: med

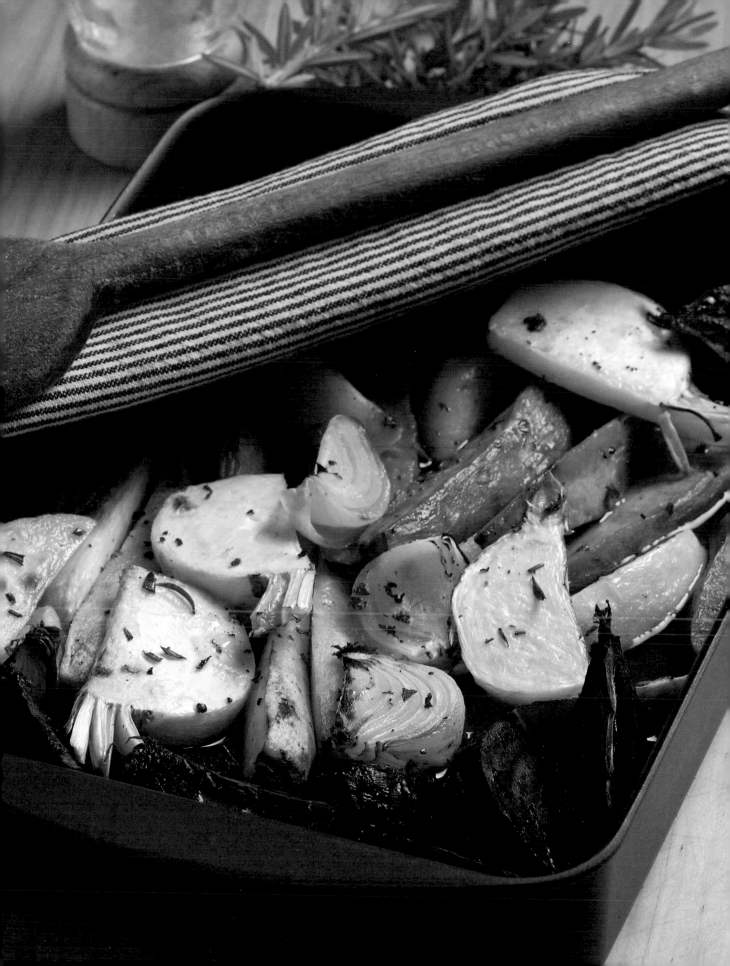

Balanced eating: protein

Recipes high in protein have been grouped together as:

- Meatless dishes: eggs, tofu, pulses (legumes), cheese, nuts
- Fish and seafood
- Meat and poultry

Meatless dishes

There are many people who choose a vegetarian style of eating, or who regularly enjoy a meal prepared without meat. This style of cooking fits in well with the principles of healthy eating for people with diabetes. Legumes (pulses) have the advantage of providing carbohydrate as well as protein. They can also be low in fat, and are often cheaper than meat.

Eggs, tofu and cheeses are excellent sources of protein and other important nutrients, but are low in carbohydrate. The addition of cheese, creams, milk or butter adds to saturated fat so try using margarine and oil in moderation and low-fat milk and cheeses.

Nuts and seeds are useful additions to dishes for flavour and texture as well as nutrition. Although they are a good source of unsaturated fats, they are high in kilojoules and should only be used in moderation.

This section contains recipes that incorporate legumes and tofu. You will find some meatless dishes containing eggs, cheese and nuts spread throughout this book, for instance:

- Eggs: Quickes, Spanish omelette, quiches (see pages 108 and 113)
- Cheese: Spinach and ricotta cannelloni (see page 143)
- Nuts: Vegetable Loaf (page opposite); Hot Thai salad (page 212); Satay sauce (page 216)

Pulses (Legumes)

Many pulse-based dishes freeze well, so can be cooked ahead and simply reheated and served.

Plan ahead if using dried legumes as most need soaking and long, slow cooking to make them soft and digestible, which means planning ahead. They can, however, be cooked ahead of time, divided into portions and frozen, then thawed for use in quick and tasty meals.

It is easy to buy a wide range of canned or vacuum-packed pulses already cooked and ready to add to recipes.

Vegetable nut loaf

This loaf is very high in fibre, and is delicious eaten hot or cold

Serves 6
Preparation/cooking time:
1 hour

Spray oil

2 medium onions, chopped

2 sticks celery, chopped

½ green capsicum (bell pepper), chopped

3 teaspoons curry powder

1 teaspoon vegetable stock powder

½ cup cooked potato, mashed

1 cup cooked pumpkin, mashed

250g (8oz) low-fat ricotta cheese

1 cup coarsely ground cashew nuts

½ cup rolled oats

½ cup dried wholegrain breadcrumbs

1 egg, beaten

2 tablespoons chopped parsley

1 teaspoon chopped fresh thyme or ½ teaspoon dried thyme

Salt (optional) and pepper to taste

2 tablespoons sesame seeds

Method

1. Preheat oven to 180°C (350°F)
2. Spray a frying pan with oil and sauté onions, celery, capsicum and curry powder for 2–3 minutes.
3. In a bowl, combine the sautéed vegetables with the rest of the ingredients (except the sesame seeds).
4. Line a loaf tin with foil or baking paper and spray with spray oil.
5. Sprinkle sesame seeds over base of tin, and then shake tin so that seeds adhere to sides as well.
6. Spoon vegetable mixture into the tin and press down firmly and neatly.
7. Bake in oven for 40–45 minutes.
8. Remove from oven and leave to stand for five minutes before turning out. Turn onto serving dish and carefully remove foil/baking paper.
9. Finally, grill on high for three to five minutes or until the top is crisp and well browned.
10. To serve: cut loaf into thick slices.

Storage: Cover and refrigerate for up to four days.

Nutrition data per serve:
1316 kJ (314 cal), carbohydrate 20g, protein 14g, fat 19g, saturated fat 5.1g, fibre 5g, sodium 167mg
GI rating: med

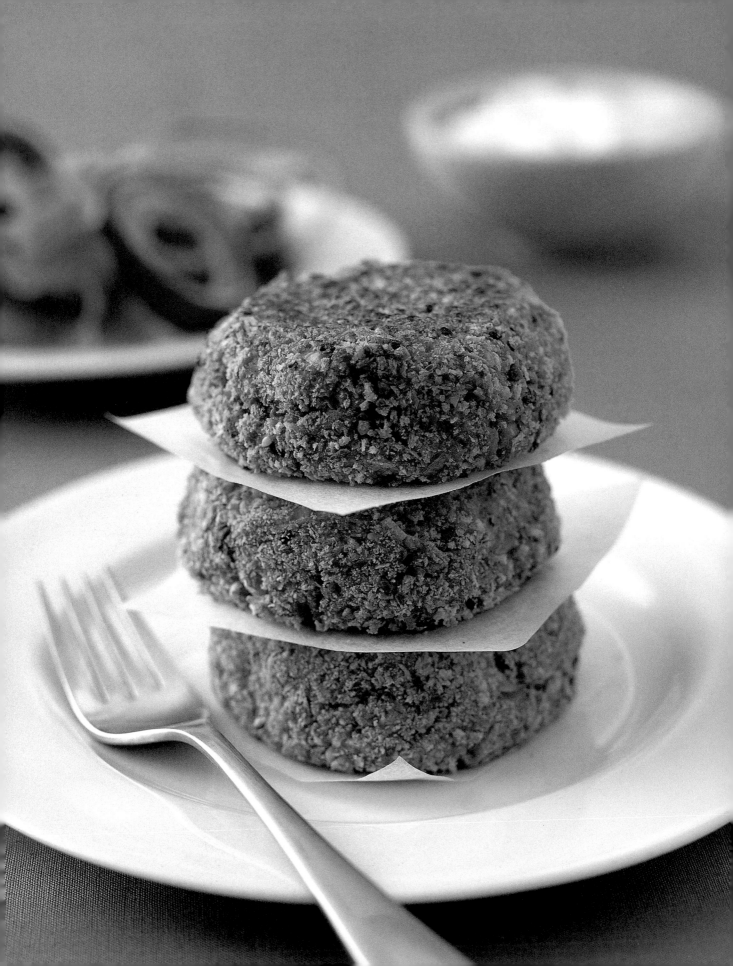

Bombay burgers with raita

Serves 4 (makes 8 patties)
Preparation/cooking time:
1 hour

1 cup dried red lentils

1 large potato, cut into pieces

1 medium onion, finely chopped

¼ cup shredded coconut

1 tablespoon sesame seeds

1 tablespoon plain flour

1 teaspoon curry powder

1 teaspoon fresh ginger

¼ teaspoon pepper

2 teaspoons lemon juice

¾–1 cup wholegrain breadcrumbs

Sliced onion rings, for garnish

1 quantity Raita (recipe below)

Method

1. Preheat oven to 190°C (375°F)
2. Rinse lentils, cover with water in a saucepan and simmer, covered, for approximately 30 minutes or until soft.
3. Add potato 10 minutes into the cooking time.
4. Drain lentils and potato, and mash thoroughly. Add onion, coconut, sesame seeds, flour, spices, grated or minced ginger and lemon juice.
5. Allow to cool (preferably chill).
6. Shape into patties and coat with breadcrumbs.
7. Bake on lightly oiled tray in oven for 10–15 minutes, or cook in a frying pan lightly sprayed with oil, taking care not to burn the coating.
8. Serve hot garnished with onion rings and accompanied with Raita (recipe follows).

Nutrition data per serve (including Raita):
1349 kJ (323 cal), carbohydrate 45g, protein 20g, fat 5g, saturated fat 1.7g, fibre 10g, sodium 162mg
GI rating: med

Raita
Serves 4
Preparation/cooking time:
30 minutes

¼ cucumber, cut in chunks

Pinch of salt (optional)

1 medium tomato, chopped

1 small onion, very finely sliced

200g (7fl oz) low-fat natural yoghurt

¼ teaspoon minced garlic

3–4 drops tabasco sauce or chilli sauce

2 tablespoons chopped mint

Method

1. Sprinkle cucumber with salt. Place in sieve over bowl and allow to drain to remove excess liquid. Place in a mixing bowl.
2. Mix tomato, onion and cucumber.
3. Mix yoghurt, garlic and tabasco or chilli sauce and the mint.
4. Pour yoghurt mixture over vegetables, mix well and refrigerate for ½ hour.
5. Serve with Bombay burgers, above.

Nutrition data per serve:
155 kJ (37 cal), carbohydrate 4g, protein 4g, fat 0g, saturated fat 0.1g, fibre 1g, sodium 42mg
GI rating: low

Mexican polenta pie

The dumplings give this already nutritious and flavoursome dish an extra carbohydrate boost. Experiment with the flavourings according to your taste for spicy food. We have suggested canned vegetables and beans to make the dish quick to prepare.

Serves 6
Preparation/cooking time:
1 hour 15 minutes

Pie:
2 teaspoons oil

1 medium onion, finely chopped

2 cloves garlic, crushed

1 green capsicum, diced

2 tablespoons no-added-salt tomato paste

400g (14oz) can whole tomatoes

400g (14oz) can corn kernels, drained

400g (14oz) can kidney beans, drained and rinsed

1 teaspoon chilli powder, or to taste

2 teaspoons Worcestershire sauce

Topping:
1 cup self-raising flour

1 cup polenta (cornmeal)

¾ cup skim milk

2 eggs, lightly beaten

1 cup grated low-fat tasty or block cheese

2 tablespoons chopped chives

Method

1. Preheat oven to 200°C (400°F)

2. Heat oil in the saucepan over medium heat and then sauté onion, garlic and capsicum for approximately three minutes until just tender.

3. Add tomato paste and tomatoes, vegetables and beans, spices, and Worcestershire sauce.

4. Boil, uncovered, for 10 minutes.

5. Transfer bean and vegetable mixture to baking dish or casserole.

6. Make the dumplings by combining the flour, cornmeal, milk, eggs, cheese and chives. Drop spoonfuls of dumpling mixture on top of the bean mixture.

7. Bake, uncovered, in oven for 10 minutes, then reduce heat to 180°C (350°F) and bake for a further 30 minutes. Serve hot.

Nutrition data per serve:
1728 kJ (413 cal), carbohydrate 60g, protein 22g, fat 7g, saturated fat 2.0g, fibre 10g, sodium 564mg
GI rating: low

Red curry of bean curd and beans

The fish sauce gives a depth of flavour to this dish but is very high in sodium.
If you need to reduce your sodium intake, it may be omitted.

Serves 4
Preparation/cooking time:
10 minutes

1 cup green beans

1 cup button mushrooms

3 medium tomatoes, chopped

400g (14oz) firm tofu (soybean curd)

2 cups low-fat evaporated milk and
1 teaspoon coconut essence
or 2 cups coconut flavoured low-fat
evaporated milk

1 tablespoon red curry paste

2 teaspoons dark brown sugar

4 lime leaves

2 red chillies, de-seeded
and sliced

Coriander leaves, for garnish

2 tablespoons fish sauce (optional)
adds a depth of flavour but is high
in sodium (salt). If using, add
at Step 3.

Method

1. Trim and slice the green beans. Slice the mushrooms and roughly chop the tomatoes.
2. Cut the tofu into 2-centimetre (¾-inch) cubes.
3. Place milk, essence, curry paste, sugar and lime leaves in a wok or saucepan. Stir and simmer for two minutes.
4. Add the mushrooms, green beans and tofu and simmer gently for another four to five minutes.
5. Remove lime leaves, stir in the sliced chillies.
6. Serve garnished with the coriander leaves.

Nutrition data per serve:
1253 kJ (300 cal), carbohydrate 21g, protein 25g, fat 12g, saturated fat 3.1g, fibre 5g, sodium 341mg
GI rating: low

Tofu sukiyaki

Serves 4, 372g per serve
Preparation/cooking time:
12 minutes

1 cup vegetable stock

400g (14oz) firm tofu,
cut into 2cm cubes

¼ cup mirin (or rice wine)

1 tablespoon brown sugar

1 tablespoon light soy sauce

4 baby bok choy, cut into quarters

1 cup thinly sliced carrots

1 cup green beans, trimmed and
diagonally sliced

1 cup mushrooms, thinly sliced

4 spring onions, diagonally sliced

Method

1. Pour stock into wok and heat until just simmering.
2. Add tofu and simmer gently for one minute.
3. With a slotted spoon gently lift tofu from wok; set aside.
4. Add mirin, sugar and soy to remaining stock in wok, stir to dissolve sugar and simmer for three minutes to reduce sauce.
5. Add bok choy, carrots, beans and mushrooms and cook for about two minutes or until they are just tender.
6. Add spring onions, return tofu to wok and gently combine with the other ingredients, being careful not to break up the tofu.
7. Serve with rice noodles or rice.

Nutrition data per serve:
752 kJ (180 cal), carbohydrate 9g, protein 15g, fat 7g, saturated fat 1.1g, fibre 5g, sodium 408mg
GI rating: low

Spinach pie

Serves 6
Preparation/cooking time:
60 minutes (including time to
make filling)

1 quantity Spinach and ricotta
filling (see page 140)

250g (9oz) extra spinach

Spray oil

8 sheets fresh filo pastry

2 teaspoons sesame seeds

1½ quantity of Orange and
cucumber salad (page 208)

Method

1. Preheat oven to 180°C (350°F)
2. Lay the pastry out on a clean dry bench.
3. Using a fairly shallow baking dish, spray this with oil, then lay one sheet over the surface—some will hang over the side.
4. Repeat this with 5 more sheets, spraying each sheet with oil. You should have pastry hanging over each side.
5. Combine the extra spinach with the Spinach and ricotta filling and spread evenly in the dish.
6. Start to cover the filling with the pastry sheets that are hanging over the sides, spraying each one lightly with oil as you go.
7. When all sheets have been folded over the filling, add one extra sheet folded to fit the top, spray with oil and place the last sheet over in the same way. Spray the top with oil, then sprinkle the sesame seeds over and bake for 35–40 minutes. The top should be golden brown and crisp.
8. Serve with Orange and cucumber salad.

Spinach pie will freeze—you will need to re-heat in a moderate oven so the pastry becomes crisp again.

> **Nutrition data per serve:**
> 1190 kJ (285 cal), carbohydrate 23g, protein 19g, fat 11g, saturated fat 5.7g, fibre 7g, sodium 443mg
> **GI rating:** med

Gado Gado

The vegetables in gado gado can be changed according to season or taste.

Serves 4
Preparation/cooking time:
30 minutes

1 cup bean shoots

1 cup green beans, trimmed

1½ cups broccoli florets

1 cup carrot rings

1 cup cabbage, diced

1 medium green capsicum, diced

6–10 snow peas

2 onions, cut into wedges

2 tomatoes, cut into wedges

1 small cucumber, peeled
and diced

4 hard-boiled eggs,
cut into quarters

1 quantity Satay sauce,
(see page 216)

Method

1. Half fill a medium saucepan with water and bring to a rapid boil.
2. Plunge the vegetables, except the tomatoes and cucumber, one variety at a time, into the boiling water for no more than one minute, or until the colour intensifies. Quickly remove the blanched vegetables from the water, place in the colander and immediately flush with cold, running water. (This preserves the colour and crispness.) Bring water back to the boil before blanching each type of vegetable. Alternatively, microwave vegetables with 2 tablespoons water on 'high' for two minutes.
3. Arrange all the ingredients on a platter with the eggs on top as garnish. Serve at either room temperature or chilled, with cooked rice and a bowl of warm satay sauce.

Storage: Cover and refrigerate for no more than one day.

Nutrition data per serve:
632 kJ (149 cal), carbohydrate 10g, protein 12g, fat 5g, saturated fat 1.6g, fibre 7g, sodium 113mg
GI rating: low

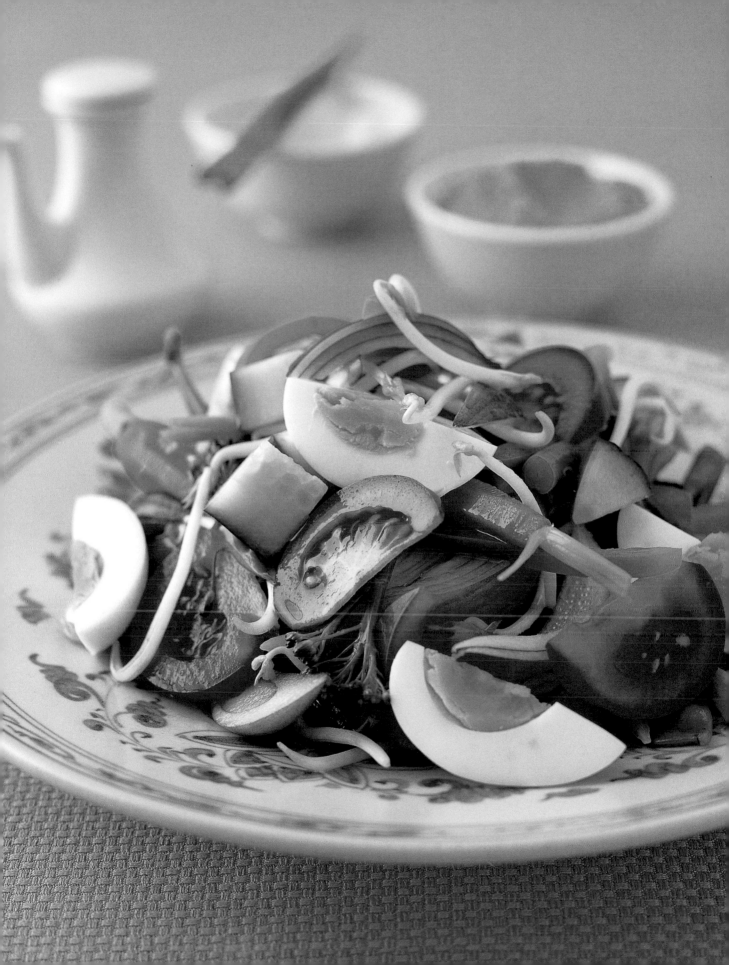

Fish and seafood

Serve fish and seafood with three serves of cooked vegetables and/or salad. For ideas see pages 199–205 for vegetables and pages 206–214 for salads. Starchy vegetables, pasta, rice or wholegrain bread can be added to make the following dishes a complete meal.

Piquant fish in foil

This is a wonderful way to prepare fresh fish. Serve it with jacket potatoes and a crisp salad.

Serves 4
Preparation/cooking time:
30–40 minutes

4 large fillets of white-fleshed fish (e.g. sea perch or barracouta), or small whole fish (e.g. whiting or bream)

2 teaspoons finely chopped fresh tarragon (or ½ teaspoon dried tarragon)

1 tablespoon very finely chopped parsley

Coarsely ground black pepper, to taste

1 medium onion, thinly sliced

1 lemon, thinly sliced

Juice of 1 lemon

2 tablespoons dry white wine

Method

1. Preheat oven to 180°C (350°F)
2. Lightly grease, or spray with non-stick cooking spray, four pieces of foil large enough to completely wrap the fish fillets.
3. Place the fish fillets on the pieces of foil. Sprinkle each fillet with the herbs and black pepper. Arrange several onion rings on top of each fillet and top with one or two slices of lemon.
4. Mix lemon juice and white wine and pour over the fish.
5. Wrap each fillet in foil, sealing along the top, so that the juices aren't lost during cooking or when opening the foil.
6. Place the foil parcels, sealed side up, on a baking tray. Bake in oven or barbecue over glowing coals for 30 minutes.
7. Open foil along the sealing edge and serve immediately.

Nutrition data per serve:
766 kJ (183 cal), carbohydrate 2g, protein 33g, fat 4g, saturated fat 1.1g, fibre 1g, sodium 144mg

Cajun fish

This is quite a spicy dish, so use less of the spice if you don't like really hot food

Serves 4
Preparation/cooking time:
15 minutes

4 pieces firm-fleshed fish

2 tablespoons cajun spice mixture
(available from supermarkets)

2 tablespoons plain flour

Spray oil

Method

1. Heat a barbecue plate or griller until really hot—it should be smoking hot.
2. Skin the fish if necessary, then coat each piece of fish well with the spice mixture mixed with the flour.
3. Spray the hot plate with oil, then place the fish on the hot surface.
4. Cook the fish on one side for two to three minutes, depending on the thickness of the fish, then turn over and cook on the other side for one to two minutes, or until just cooked. The surface of the fish will be black.
5. Serve the fish with jacket potatoes and salad (eg Spinach Valentino), or rice (see recipes), or a bed of stir-fried vegetables, accompanied by lemon or lime wedges.

Nutrition data per serve:
775 kJ (185 cal), carbohydrate 4g, protein 33g, fat 4g,
saturated fat 1.2g, fibre trace, sodium 138mg

Fish in orange sauce

Serves 4
Preparation/cooking time:
15 minutes

Juice of 2 oranges

Juice of 1 lemon

1 teaspoon margarine

¼ teaspoon black pepper, coarsely ground

4 fillets fish

Small quantity of plain flour

Method

1. Place juices, margarine and pepper in pan.
2. Cook until slightly reduced.
3. Dust fish with flour.
4. Add to sauce and poach until just cooked, turning once.
5. Lift out onto serving plates. Spoon sauce over the fish.

Nutrition data per serve:
824 kJ (197 cal), carbohydrate 5g, protein 33g, fat 5g, saturated fat 1.3g, fibre trace, sodium 150mg

Whole fish in ginger

Serves 4
Preparation/cooking time:
40 minutes

1kg (2lb) whole fish (e.g. snapper, blue eye or coral trout), gutted and scaled, but with head intact

2 teaspoons chopped or minced fresh ginger

1 clove garlic, crushed

2 tablespoons light soy sauce

Juice of 1 lemon

¾ cup dry white wine

4 spring onions, sliced lengthways

Lemon slices, for garnish

Method

1. Using a very sharp knife, score the skin of the fish on each side, three or four times, at equal intervals and at an angle to the backbone.
2. Place fish on its side in a flat dish, or support it upright with wooden skewers.
3. Combine remaining ingredients to make a marinade, and pour over the fish.
4. Bake the fish, uncovered, in a 180°C (350°F) oven for 30 minutes or until fish flakes when tested with a fork.
5. Baste frequently with the marinade during cooking. Alternatively, cover with plastic film and microwave on high for 15 minutes.
6. Serve the fish whole with cooking juices, garnished with lemon slices.

Nutrition data per serve:
727kJ (174 cal), carbohydrate 2g, protein 27g, fat 3g, saturated fat 0.9g, fibre 1g, sodium 490mg

Salmon mornay

Serves 6
Preparation/cooking time:
50 minutes

440g (15½oz) salmon, canned in water, drained

6 spring onions, chopped

2 tablespoons lemon juice

2 stalks celery, finely chopped

2 tablespoons chopped parsley

2 hard-boiled eggs, chopped

Pepper and salt (optional) to taste

Paprika

1 quantity Cheese sauce (see page 216)

½ cup dry wholegrain breadcrumbs

½ teaspoon dried mixed herbs

Method

1. Preheat the oven to 180°C (350°F)
2. Drain the salmon, removing black skin and bones. Break salmon into pieces (not too small) and place in a mixing bowl.
3. Add the spring onions, lemon juice, celery, chopped eggs, parsley and pepper and salt to taste.
4. Pour the cheese sauce over salmon mixture.
5. Fold together carefully to avoid breaking up the salmon too much.
6. Spoon into a shallow casserole dish.
7. Combine breadcrumbs with the herbs and sprinkle over the top.
8. Bake in oven for 30 minutes. Alternatively, cover and microwave on medium for 12–14 minutes, and stand, covered, for 5 minutes before serving.
9. Sprinkle with a little paprika to serve.

Nutrition data per serve:
1096kJ (262 cal), carbohydrate 13g, protein 27g, fat 11g, saturated fat 3.5g, fibre 2g, sodium 298mg
GI rating: low

Curried tuna
and rice casserole

The tuna in this recipe can be replaced with red or pink salmon.

Serves 4
Preparation/cooking time:
1 hour 40 minutes

425g (15oz) tuna, canned
in water, drained

Juice of 1 lemon

120g (4oz) Mahatma™ white long
grain or basmati rice

2 small onions, diced

2–3 teaspoons curry powder

2 tablespoons flour

3 cups skim (or reduced fat) milk

Salt (optional) and pepper to taste

2 slices wholegrain bread,
crumbled

Method

1. Preheat the oven to 160°C (325°F)

2. Mix tuna and lemon juice in a bowl.

3. Cook rice in boiling water, or microwave.

4. Drain rice and combine with the tuna mixture.

5. Dry fry onion and curry powder in a saucepan.

6. Combine flour with a little of the milk to make a smooth
   runny mixture.

7. Add remaining milk to onions and curry powder and bring to
   the boil. Remove from heat and add the flour paste.

8. Return to heat and stir continually until mixture thickens.
   Check flavour—add pepper and/or salt if needed.

9. Pour two-thirds of the curry sauce over tuna and rice. Mix.

10. Spoon into a casserole and pour the remaining sauce over
    the top.

11. Cover with breadcrumbs, and bake in oven until golden and
    the casserole is heated through (approximately 30 minutes).

Storage: cover and refrigerate for 24 hours.

Nutrition data per serve:
1436 kJ (434 cal), carbohydrate 44g, protein 33g, fat 3g, saturated
fat 1.2g, fibre 2g, sodium 218mg
GI rating: low–med

Pasta marinara

Serves 4
Preparation/cooking time:
20 minutes + 20 minutes for
tomato sauce

1 quantity Fresh tomato sauce
(see page 139)

300g (10½oz) pasta (e.g.
spaghetti, tagliatelle or pasta
of choice)

500g (1lb) seafood marinara mix
(fresh or frozen)

Spray oil

1 tablespoon chopped parsley

Method

1. Make 1 quantity fresh tomato sauce and set aside to keep warm.
2. Fill a large saucepan two-thirds full with water, and bring to a rapid boil. Add pasta, and boil rapidly for 10–12 minutes until al dente (tender, but still firm to bite), drain and set aside.
3. While the pasta is cooking, add the seafood to large frying pan sprayed lightly with oil, toss until cooked through—this only takes a few minutes. Add the tomato sauce to the seafood, check flavour and adjust to your taste (you may wish to add more garlic or freshly ground black pepper).
4. Add the pasta to the sauce. Toss gently to combine. Sprinkle with parsley and serve immediately.

Nutrition date per serve:
1822 kJ (436 cal), carbohydrate 57g, protein 31g, fat 6g, saturated fat 1.1g, fibre 5g, sodium 392mg
GI rating: low

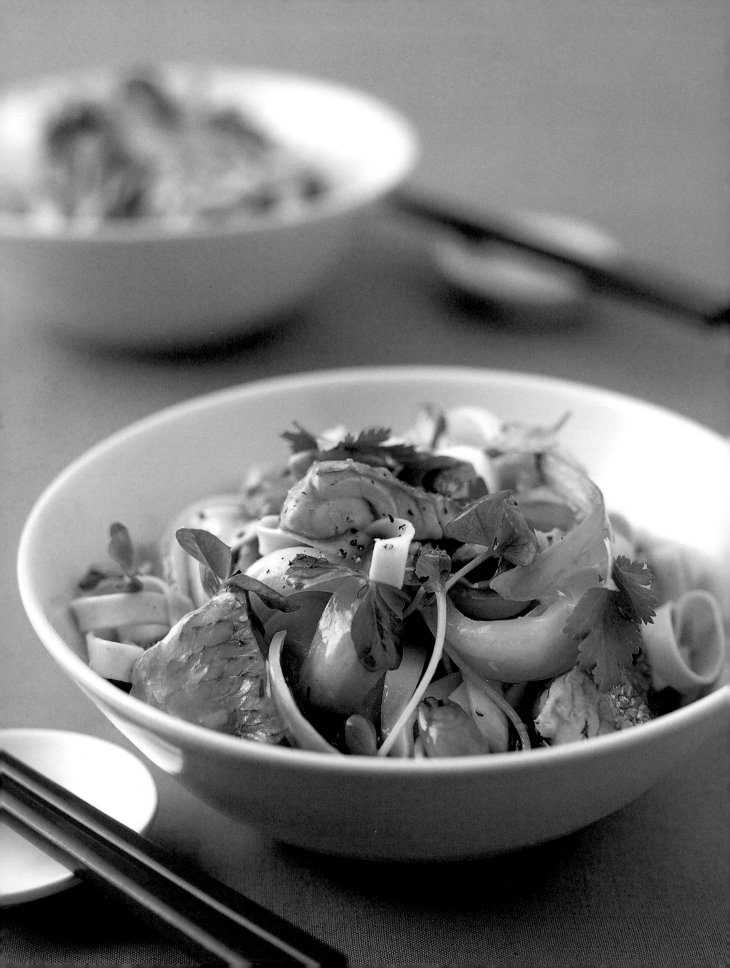

Stir-fried bok choy
with fish and almonds

For variety, all or part of the fish can be replaced with scallops, chicken, or tofu.

Serves 4
Preparation/cooking time:
30 minutes

4 fillets white-fleshed fish (e.g. snapper or flathead), cut into bite-sized pieces

2 teaspoons finely chopped or minced fresh ginger

2 tablespoons chopped fresh coriander

1 lemon, juice and grated rind

3 tablespoons teriyaki sauce

Spray oil

1 bunch baby bok choy, washed and roughly chopped

1 large Spanish (red) onion, peeled and diced

1 cup snow pea shoots or bean sprouts

Black pepper

Salt (optional)

200g (7oz) fresh rice noodles, cooked

70g (2oz) toasted almonds, for garnish

4 sprigs coriander, for garnish

Method

1. Marinate fish in ginger, coriander, lemon juice, rind and teriyaki sauce for 15 minutes.
2. Spray wok with oil, add fish and marinade and bring to boil.
3. Reduce to simmer, add bok choy and onion and stir-fry for about two minutes or until greens are just tender but still brightly coloured.
4. Add snow pea shoots or bean sprouts and continue to stir-fry until all ingredients are warmed through.
5. Season with black pepper to taste.
6. Add cooked noodles. Stir-fry to mix ingredients evenly until warmed through.
7. Serve on warmed plates and garnish with almonds and sprigs of coriander.

Nutrition date per serve:
1702 kJ (409 cal), carbohydrate 23g, protein 41g, fat 15g, saturated fat 2g, fibre 5g, sodium 284mg
GI rating: low

Salmon and potato cakes

These patties can be served in toasted grainy bread rolls with lettuce and sliced tomato as fish burgers. The patties also make a tasty topping for toasted bread or cold as a sandwich filling.

Serves 4 (2 cakes per person)
Preparation/cooking time:
45 minutes

500g (1lb) potato, peeled and roughly cut (makes about 2 cups mash)

400g (14oz) pink or red salmon, canned in water, drained, skin and bones removed

1 red onion, peeled and chopped very fine

2 teaspoons grated lemon or lime rind

1 teaspoon chopped lemon thyme, lemon grass, or ½ teaspoon dried lemon myrtle

2 tablespoons lemon juice

2 tablespoons chopped fresh parsley

1 egg, lightly beaten

Salt and pepper to taste (optional)

½–¾ cup dried wholegrain breadcrumbs

1 tablespoons oil for cooking—or omit and bake the salmon cakes in the oven

Method

1. Cook the potato until tender, drain and mash, chill in refrigerator 15 minutes (even better if cooked ahead of time and chilled).
2. Combine the salmon, onion, rind, herbs, lemon juice in a mixing bowl.
3. Add the potato, egg, salt and pepper if needed, blend well.
4. Divide into 8 portions, then shape into patties and toss in the crumbs, pressing the crumbs into the patties.
5. Fry in the hot oil until brown, turn and cook on the other side until brown or place the patties on a baking tray covered with baking paper, spray both sides of each patty lightly with the oil, bake until brown—about 15–20 minutes in a preheated oven at 180°C (350°F)
6. Serve with salad or cooked vegetables.

Note: this can be served with a wedge of lemon, a spoonful of light mayonnaise, or make a tasty dressing by combining 2 tablespoons low-fat mayonnaise with 2 teaspoons hoi sin sauce, 1–2 teaspoons sweet chilli sauce, and 1 teaspoon sugar—mix well together. This serves 4 people.

Nutrition data per serve:
13g1427 kJ (341cal), carbohydrate 24g, protein 29g, fat 13g, saturated fat 2.7g, fibre 4g, sodium 191mg
GI rating: high

Homemade fish and chips

Fish and chips are thought to be best if eaten occasionally as a treat, rather than a regular meal, because of the high fat content. This version is quite low in fat, easy to prepare, and everyone will love it! Remember that fish only takes a short time to cook.

Serves 4
Preparation/cooking time:
45 minutes

Chips:
800g (1¾lb) potatoes
(choose a variety labelled as good
for making chips if you can)

Spray oil

Seasoning to your taste,
e.g., pepper and salt, dried herbs,
a little Cajun seasoning

Fish:
500g (1lb) fresh or frozen firm
fleshed fish—flathead, dory,
whiting etc

1 egg

2 tablespoons water

1 tablespoon plain flour

1 cup seasoned breadcrumbs
(use commercial seasoned
crumbs or make your own by
adding salt and pepper and dried
herbs to breadcrumbs)

1 tablespoon oil

Method

1. Preheat oven to 200°C (400°F)
2. Peel potatoes, cut into chips or wedges, microwave until just tender (about 4 minutes), drain.
3. Spray with oil, add spices and toss gently to coat potatoes.
4. Spread chips on an oven tray covered with baking paper, making sure they are well spread out, place in oven and bake until brown and crispy—allow 30–40 minutes, turning over once during the cooking. If you have a fan-forced oven, use this facility to help make chips crisper.
5. While the potatoes are cooking, prepare the fish.
6. Beat egg with the water.
7. Place flour and crumbs in separate shallow dishes.
8. Coat each piece of fish with flour, dip into the egg mixture, then coat in crumbs and place the fish on a tray or plate.
9. About 10 minutes before the chips are ready, heat the oil in a large frying pan, add the fish, and cook quickly on fairly high heat for 2–3 minutes, then turn over and cook on the other side for 2–3 minutes. Check by inserting a sharp knife into the centre of one piece—it should be white and firm to touch.
10. Serve the fish and chips with a wedge of lemon and a crisp salad.

Nutrition data per serve:
1881 kJ (449 cal), carbohydrate 49g, protein 36g, fat 10g, saturated fat 2.2g, fibre 5g, sodium 342mg
GI rating: high

Thai fish cakes

If your family find these too spicy replace the chilli with 2 teaspoons of sweet chilli sauce.
These fish cakes are suitable for a light meal or lunch and make a finger or party food.
Use the recipe to make 20 bite-size patties.

Serves four: 12 fish cakes
Preparation/cooking time:
20 minutes

300g (10½oz) fresh white fish fillets without skin and bones

1 egg

2 tablespoon cornflour

2 teaspoon red curry paste

2 spring onions, finely chopped

4 green beans, finely sliced

½ small hot red chilli, seeded and finely chopped

¼ cup fresh coriander, finely chopped

2 teaspoons oil

4 tablespoons Hot Thai dressing (page 220) as dipping sauce

Method

1. Place fish, egg, cornflour and curry paste and into a food processor and blend until smooth.
2. Place in bowl and add onion, beans, chilli and coriander. Mix well.
3. Form into 12 even sized patties using two wet soup spoons.
4. Heat oil in a non-stick pan and cook fish cakes each side until a golden brown and cooked through.
5. Serve with Hot Thai dressing.

Note: This recipe is high in sodium (salt). Use only occcasionally.

Nutrition data per serve:
680 kJ (163 cal), carbohydrate 7g, protein 18g, fat 6g, saturated fat 1.3g, fibre 1g, sodium 750mg
GI rating: med

Poultry and meat

Meat and poultry provide many important nutrients but may be high in saturated fats. Serve meat and poultry with three serves of cooked vegetables and/or salad. For ideas see pages 199–205 for vegetables and pages 206–214 for salads. Starchy vegetables, pasta, rice on wholegrain bread can be added to make the following dishes a complete meal.

Chicken enchiladas

Don't try storing the enchiladas, they will become soggy. You should serve them immediately they are heated through. Heat them in the oven, not in the microwave.
Corn tortillas give an authentic flavour to this Mexican dish but soft flour tortillas may also be used.

Serves 4
Preparation/cooking time:
1 hour

2 cups cooked, chopped skinless chicken breast

1 large onion, finely chopped

8–10 drops tabasco sauce or to taste

¼ teaspoon salt (optional)

¼ teaspoon ground black pepper

8 corn or soft flour tortillas, suitable for enchiladas

2 cups fresh, tomato, pureed or canned, no-added-salt tomato puree

Additional Tabasco sauce to taste

½ cup grated low-fat tasty or block cheese

1 ripe avocado

Juice ½ lemon

Method

1. Combine chicken and onion in a mixing bowl.
2. Add Tabasco sauce, and salt and pepper to chicken mixture. Mix well. Taste and adjust seasoning.
3. Preheat tortillas in oven or microwave to soften.
4. Wrap each tortilla around one eighth of chicken mixture.
5. Pack into casserole or baking dish.
6. Combine tomato puree with tabasco sauce, and pour over chicken rolls.
7. Sprinkle with cheese.
8. Bake in a preheated 200°C (400°F) oven until rolls are heated through and cheese has melted.
9. Peel avocado and remove stone. Mash flesh in a separate bowl with lemon juice.
10. Spoon a little avocado mixture over each serving.

Storage: Not suitable to store.

Nutrition data per serve:
1547 kJ (370 cal), carbohydrate 21g, protein 25g, fat 19g, saturated fat 5g, fibre 5g, sodium 214mg
GI rating: med

Tandoori chicken

Serves 4
Preparation/cooking time:
1 hour 15 minutes + 1 hour
marinating time

½ cup low-fat yoghurt

2 tablespoons tandoori paste

2 teaspoons lemon juice

1 teaspoon minced/grated ginger

2 teaspoons sugar

4 skinless chicken breasts

Method

1. Preheat oven to 150°C (300°F)
2. Fold tandoori paste, lemon juice ginger and sugar into yoghurt.
3. Coat chicken breasts in yoghurt mixture and allow to stand for at least one hour.
4. Place in shallow casserole, cover with lid or aluminium foil, and bake for one hour in oven until tender.

Nutrition data per serve:
986 kJ (236 cal), carbohydrate 5g, protein 29g, fat 11g, saturated fat 2.5g, fibre 1g, sodium 478mg
GI rating: low

Apricot chicken

Serves 4
Preparation/cooking time:
40 minutes

2 cups solid-pack canned apricots

4 skinless chicken breasts

1 large onion, coarsely chopped

Ground black pepper, to taste

2 sage leaves, finely chopped
or ½ teaspoon dried sage

1 sprig thyme, chopped

2 tablespoons fruit chutney

1 tablespoon cornflour
(cornstarch)

3 tablespoons water

1 tablespoon finely chopped
chives or mint, for garnish

Method

1. Preheat oven to 180°C (350°F)
2. Reserve four apricot halves for garnish. Puree remaining apricots.
3. Arrange chicken fillets in a single layer in a casserole, and sprinkle onion, pepper and herbs over the top.
4. Combine chutney and apricot puree and pour over the chicken. Bake in oven for 30 minutes.
5. Mix the cornflour and water to a smooth consistency.
6. Remove casserole from oven and drain.
7. Drain the sauce from the casserole into a saucepan.
8. Add the cornflour and water to the sauce and heat, stirring constantly, until it thickens. Cook a further two minutes.
9. Arrange a chicken breast on each plate and spoon sauce over. Garnish with apricot halves and chopped chives.

Nutrition data per serve:
1088 kJ (260 cal), carbohydrate 18g, protein 28g, fat 7g, saturated fat 2.1g, fibre 3g, sodium 125mg
GI rating: med

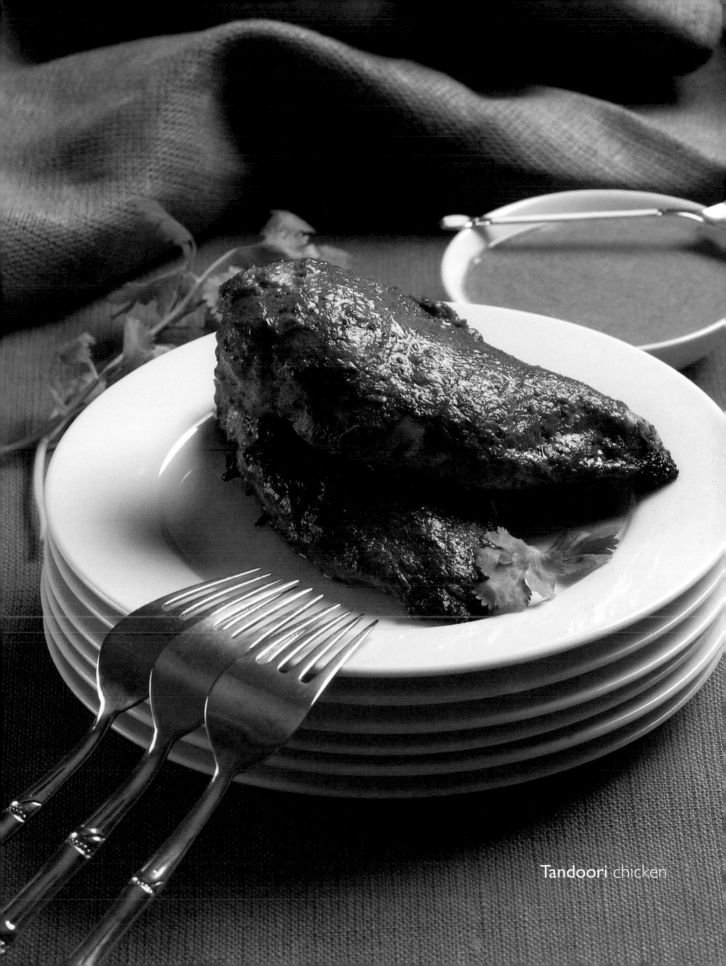

Tandoori chicken

Satay chicken

This Malaysian recipe makes a great alternative for the barbecue.
Green prawns, pork, beef or lamb fillet are all delicious flavoured with this marinade.

Serves 4 (3 skewers each)
Preparation/cooking time:
1 hour 30 minutes

500g (1lb) chicken fillets

1 clove garlic, crushed

2 tablespoons light soy sauce

2 tablespoons lemon juice

1 small onion, grated

1 teaspoon oil

1 quantity of Satay sauce to serve
(see page 216)

Method

1. Soak 12 wooden skewers in water for at least an hour, to prevent them burning on the barbecue.
2. Cut chicken into small cubes or strips.
3. Thread the chicken onto skewers. Arrange the skewers on a flat dish.
4. Combine remaining ingredients and brush over the chicken. Leave chicken to marinate for at least an hour, turning occasionally.
5. Grill or barbecue the satay chicken, turning frequently and basting from time to time with marinade.
6. Serve hot, accompanied by satay sauce.

Storage: Use on day of preparation. However, the dish may be made some hours ahead of time and kept, covered, in the refrigerator. You can freeze uncooked satay.

Nutrition data per serve:
1431 kJ (342 cal), carbohydrate 5g, protein 31g, fat 21g, saturated fat 5.1g, fibre 3g, sodium 650mg

Green pork curry

Instead of coconut milk, this recipe uses low-fat evaporated skim milk and coconut essence or coconut flavoured low-fat evaporated milk—a great way to reduce the fat content!

Serves 4
Preparation/cooking time:
35 minutes

1–2 tablespoons low-fat commercial green curry paste

1½ tablespoons cornflour (cornstarch)

1 cup low-fat evaporated milk and ¾ teaspoon coconut essence

or 1 cups coconut flavoured low-fat evaporated milk

500g (1lb) lean pork fillet, cut into bite-sized pieces

200g (7oz) French beans, trimmed and halved

1 red capsicum, de-seeded and diced

250g (8½oz) bean sprouts

Sprigs of fresh basil or coriander (optional)

Method

1. Mix cornflour with a little evaporated milk to form a smooth paste, add remaining evaporated milk and coconut essence and set aside.
2. Spray wok with cooking oil and sauté pork until tender and just beginning to brown; set aside.
3. Add curry paste, beans and capsicum to wok and toss for about two minutes.
4. Add cornflour and milk mixture and stir until sauce thickens and cooks.
5. Add bean sprouts and pork and stir until heated through.
6. Serve on bed of rice or noodles, garnished with the basil or coriander leaves.

Nutrition data per serve:
1091 kJ (261 cal), carbohydrate 14g, protein 36g, fat 6g, saturated fat 1.4g, fibre 4g, sodium 327mg
GI rating: low

Pork with mango

This is a great recipe that is very easy to prepare and yet looks and tastes good enough for a special occasion. Add simple boiled rice and a crisp green salad to round out the meal. You can substitute chicken if you wish.

Serves 4
Preparation/cooking time:
40 minutes

2 small or 1 large mango

1 cup dry white wine

3 tablespoons mango chutney

4 tablespoons chopped spring onions

4 lean pork schnitzels or butterfly pork steaks

A little plain flour

Spray oil

2 tablespoons water

4 spring onions, for garnish

Method

1. Make the sauce: peel the mangoes, cut away and roughly slice the flesh.
2. Place the mango flesh in a saucepan. Add the white wine and chutney.
3. Bring to the boil, reduce heat and simmer until the sauce has reduced by half, about 15 minutes.
4. If you want a smooth sauce, puree the hot fruit mixture in a food processor or blender, or force through a sieve. Return to saucepan.
5. Add the chopped spring onions. Return to the boil.
6. Reduce heat and simmer for a further two to three minutes.
7. Dust the schnitzels with the plain flour. While the sauce is simmering, brush or spray a large frying pan with oil and heat over medium-high heat.
8. Fry the schnitzels, turning occasionally, for approximately 10 minutes until browned on both sides.
9. Remove the cooked schnitzels from the pan. Add the 2 tablespoons of water to the pan, as well as the sauce. Heat, stirring constantly, for about three minutes.
10. Arrange the schnitzels on individual dinner plates. Spoon the sauce over the schnitzels and garnish with the whole spring onions.

Nutrition data per serve:
1175 kJ (281 cal), carbohydrate 18g, protein 29g, fat 5g, saturated fat 1.7g, fibre 2g, sodium 222mg
GI rating: med

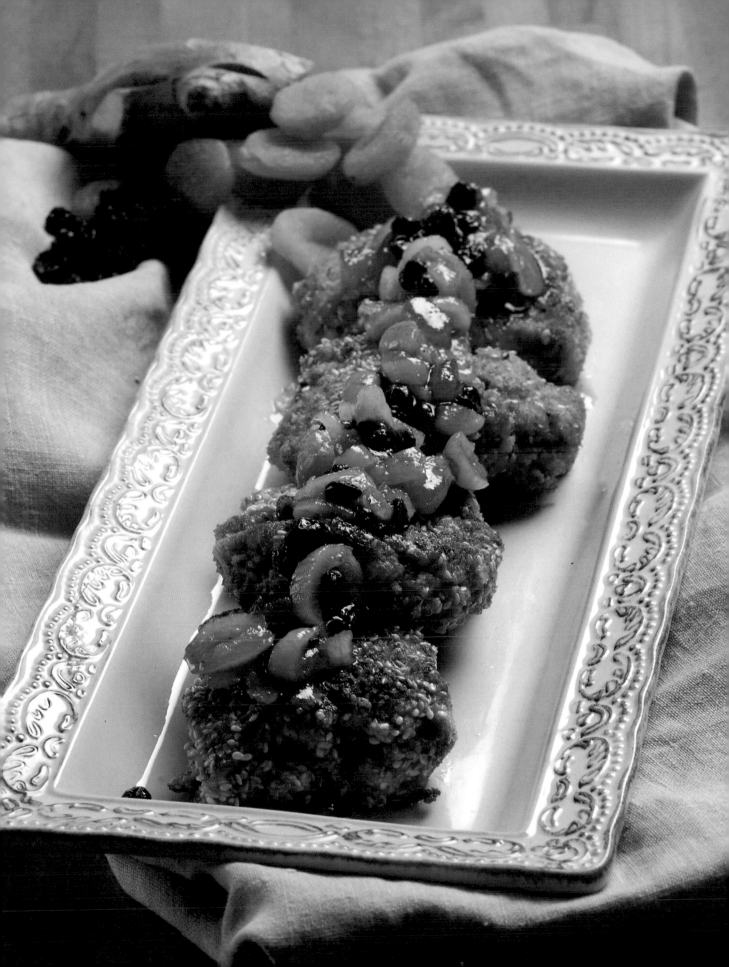

Apricot and sesame pork

This is a wonderful recipe. The brandy loses its alcohol during heating, but rounds out the lovely fruity sauce. Leave it out if you prefer.

Serves 4
Preparation/cooking time:
1 hour

1 cup boiling water

½ cup dried apricots

2 tablespoons dried currants

500g (1lb) pork scotch fillet, trimmed of fat

1 beaten egg

2 tablespoons sesame seeds

2 tablespoons dried breadcrumbs

1 clove garlic, finely chopped or minced (optional)

2 tablespoons mango chutney

1 tablespoon brandy (optional)

¼ cup canned evaporated skim milk

Method

1. Preheat oven to 200ºC (400ºF)

2. Pour boiling water over apricots and currants in a bowl, and set aside for half an hour.

3. Roll pork first in egg and then in the mixture of sesame seeds, breadcrumbs and garlic until well coated. Pat the mixture firmly onto the meat.

4. Place in roasting pan and bake, uncovered, in the oven for 45 minutes.

5. While meat is cooking, heat apricots in a saucepan with the currants and the water in which they were soaked. Simmer gently until water is almost absorbed.

6. Add chutney and brandy and stir until the sauce returns to the simmer.

7. Pour evaporated skim milk in a heat-resistant bowl and gradually stir in the hot apricot mixture (this method will prevent the milk curdling).

8. Return to saucepan and reheat without boiling.

9. To test if meat is cooked, pierce with a skewer. The juice should be clear.

10. Cut meat into eight slices, arrange two slices on each serving plate and spoon sauce over.

Variation: Substitute ½ cup of crushed pineapple for the apricots, but remember to reduce the water to ½ cup.

Storage: Both meat and sauce will keep for two days if well covered in the refrigerator. They can be served cold, in which case store meat in one piece and slice thinly just before serving, using the cold sauce as an accompaniment.

Nutrition data per serve:
1274 kJ (305 cal), carbohydrate 24 g, protein 33g, fat 8g, saturated fat 1.8g, fibre 4g, sodium 233mg
GI rating: low

Rissoles

This basic recipe can be adapted to a variety of uses. Apart from serving as rissoles with salad or vegetables, you can make hamburgers, meatballs in tomato gravy (see page 193), small meatballs served on toothpicks for parties, or made into skewers for a barbecue.

The mixture can be used to make 30 small meatballs. For barbecue or party, make the rissole mixture, divide into small portions, shape into balls with your hands, dust with flour, cook in a frying pan greased with spray oil, cooking in batches and tossing regularly so they brown on all sides. Keep warm until serving time, or make ahead of time, refrigerate, and re-heat in the oven before serving time. Serve with barbecue sauce.

**Serves 4
(8 rissoles, 2 per serve)
Preparation/cooking time:
30 minutes**

500g (1lb) lean minced beef

2 tablespoons parsley, finely chopped

½ cup dried wholegrain breadcrumbs

1 egg

1 onion, chopped finely

1 teaspoon dried mixed herbs or oregano

2 small or 1 large carrot, grated

Salt (optional) and pepper to taste

¼ cup wholemeal plain flour

Spray oil

Method

1. Place meat in a mixing bowl, add the parsley, breadcrumbs, egg, onion, herbs, carrot and pepper. Mix together really well, preferably with your hand—this helps tenderise the meat and blends flavours well, plus the rissoles hold together better if the mixture is well kneaded.
2. Place flour in a shallow dish or plate.
3. Divide the meat mixture into 8, then drop each one in the flour, dusting all over with flour, then shape into round patties, flattening them slightly as you go.
4. Spray a frying pan with oil, place rissoles in the pan, and cook, browning on one side then turning over to brown the other side—allow about 15 minutes cooking time.
5. Serve with vegetables or salad.

Nutrition data per serve (excluding raw fillings):
1248 kJ (298 cal), carbohydrate 16g, protein 31g, fat 12g, saturated fat 4.2g, fibre 3g, sodium 203mg
GI rating: low–med

Beef and bean burritos

Burritos should be eaten with the fingers. This recipe is great for a casual family meal, or for children's parties.

Serves 4 (2 tortillas per serve)
Preparation/cooking time:
2 hours

8 soft flour or corn tortillas

1 quantity Bolognese sauce (see page 138). Note changes to this recipe for tacos or burritos

400g (14oz) cooked red kidney beans, no added salt or 410g (14½oz) can red kidney beans, rinsed and drained

Shredded lettuce, finely chopped onion and tomato, slices of avocado and grated low-fat cheese, to serve

Method

1. Add kidney beans to Bolognese sauce mix and cook for a few minutes to allow flavours to blend.

2. Keep meat and bean mixture warm until tortillas are ready or allow to cool. Refrigerate and reheat when needed—this mixture also freezes well.

3. Warm tortillas, following directions on package.

4. Place some hot filling onto each tortilla, together with any combination of lettuce, onion, tomato, avocado and grated cheese, and roll up. Serve immediately.

Variation: Use Mountain bread or Pita bread as an alternative to tortillas. The snack size pita breads can be used as pockets to place the fillings into.

Nutrition data per serve (excluding raw fillings):
2111 kJ (505 cal), carbohydrate 47g, protein 44g, fat 13g, saturated fat 4.1g, fibre 17g, sodium 374mg
GI rating: low

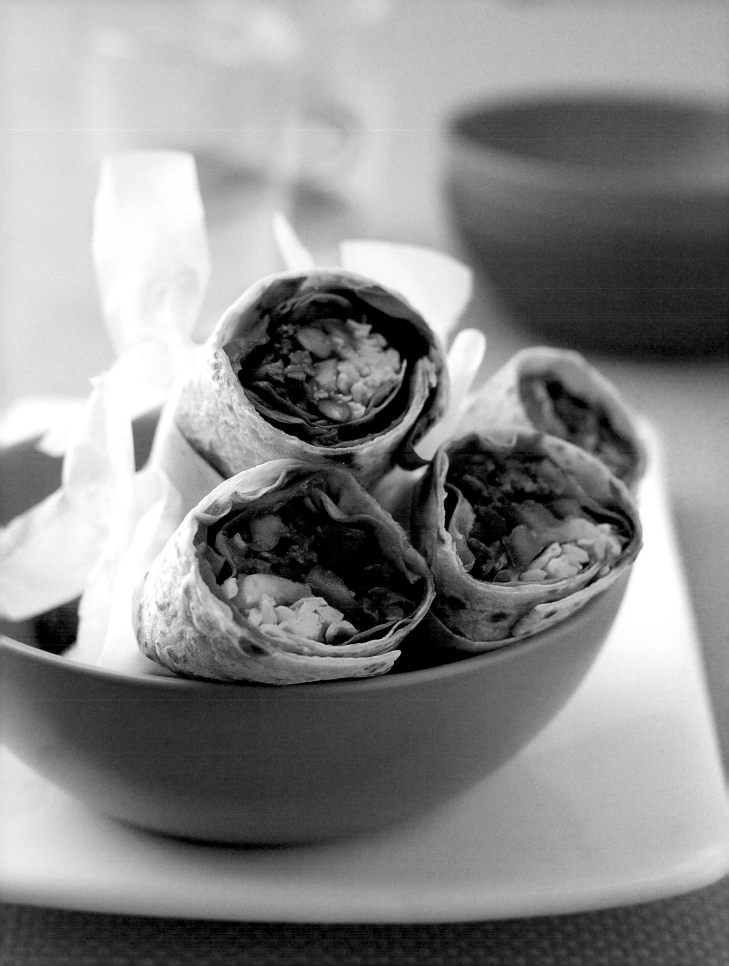

Beef curry

This dish is best when prepared the day before eating, to allow the flavour to develop.
A pinch of salt helps bring out the taste of the spices, but use sparingly.

Serves 4
Preparation/cooking time:
2–2½ hours

500g (1lb) lean beef (e.g. topside, round, bolar blade)

Ground black pepper

Spray oil (optional)

1 large onion, peeled and chopped

½ cup skinned and chopped pumpkin

1 cup peeled and chopped orange sweet potato

2 zucchini, trimmed and cut into chunks

1 tablespoon Indian curry paste (e.g. Korma)

2 teaspoons finely chopped fresh or minced ginger

½ x 400g can chickpeas

1 clove garlic, crushed

1 cup water

Pinch of salt to taste (optional)

Method

1. Preheat the oven to 200°C (400°F)
2. Trim any fat from meat. Cut into 2–3cm (1in) cubes and sprinkle with pepper.
3. In a frying pan, dry fry meat (or sauté using spray oil) until browned on all sides. Set aside in a bowl.
4. In the same frying pan, sauté the vegetables and set aside with the meat.
5. Add the curry paste to the frying pan and cook for a minute over medium heat, stirring to prevent burning, to release the fragrance, then add the ginger, garlic and chickpeas.
6. Add water and stir the pan juices well.
7. Return meat and vegetables to pan, add salt if desired, and stir to combine the flavours.
8. Spoon into a casserole, cover and cook in oven for approximately 1½–2 hours until meat is tender.
9. Serve with rice and an accompaniment such as mango chutney.

Great accompaniments to curry: Raita (see page 161), pineapple, pawpaw, sliced banana and/or diced apple, sultanas with coconut are all excellent. Poppadums (see page 249) are also delicious as part of a curry meal.

Storage: Cover and refrigerate for up to four days.

Nutrition data per serve:
1033 kJ (247 cal), carbohydrate 14g, protein 32g, fat 6g, saturated fat 2.5g, fibre 5g, sodium 204mg
GI rating: low

Italian-style beef

Although beef fillets and rumps are relatively expensive cuts of meat, you use only 500g (1lb) to feed four people. The meat cooks quickly, so there is little shrinkage. As the fillet is lean, there is no waste associated with removing excess fat.

Serves 4
Preparation/cooking time:
15 minutes

500g (1lb) lean beef fillet or rump

1 teaspoon oil

1 clove garlic, crushed

½ cup sliced mushrooms

2 large tomatoes, peeled and chopped

2 spring onions, chopped

4 leaves fresh basil, roughly chopped, or ¼ teaspoon dried basil

Freshly ground black pepper

Salt to taste (optional)

Spring onion, for garnish

Method

1. Cut the meat into thin strips, about 5-centimetres (2-inches) long and 1-centimetre (⅓-inch) wide.
2. Brush or spray oil over the base of a heavy frying pan and heat the pan over medium-high heat.
3. When hot, toss in the meat and stir-fry until well sealed and browned (approximately two to three minutes).
4. Set the meat aside on a warm plate and continue as follows: to the hot frying pan add the garlic and the mushrooms and stir-fry for a further few seconds until the mushrooms are lightly cooked.
5. Add the chopped tomatoes, spring onions, basil, pepper and salt, and bring to a simmer. Now return the meat to the sauce and simmer for about five minutes, or until the meat is cooked and the dish is hot.
6. Finally, spoon the meat and sauce onto a bed of rice or pasta, garnish with spring onion and serve.

Variation: The recipe will work just as successfully if you use veal, pork or chicken. Add a few drops of tabasco sauce if you want to make the sauce more piquant.

Storage: Cover and refrigerate for up to three days.

Nutrition data per serve:
797 kJ (191 cal), carbohydrate 3g, protein 26g, fat 7g, saturated fat 2.8g, fibre 2g, sodium 68mg

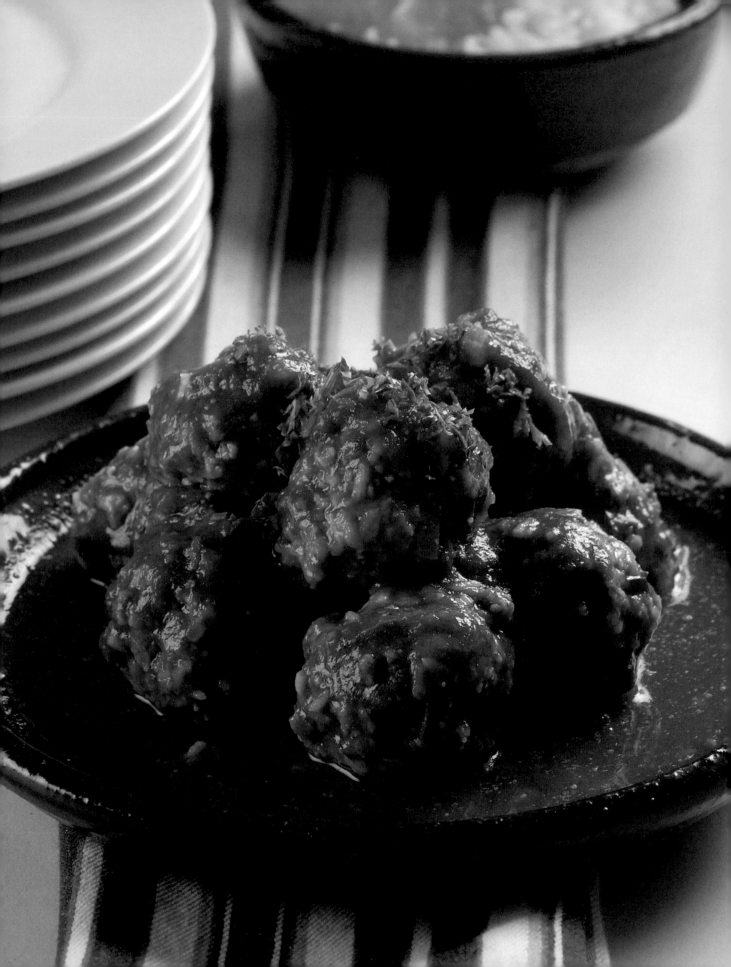

Meatballs in tomato gravy

*As the tomato mixture is acid, it helps to lower the GI of the meal especially
if you serve the meatballs with mashed potato.*

**Serves 6 (30 meatballs,
5 per serve)
Preparation/cooking time:
45 minutes**

1 quantity of rissole mixture

½ cup low-GI rice

¼ cup plain flour

400g (14oz) can concentrated
tomato soup + 1 can water
(as per tomato soup recipe)

400g (14oz) no-added-salt tomato
juice.

Chopped parsley, for garnish

Method

1. Make the rissole mixture, adding the raw rice at Step 1.
2. Place flour into a shallow dish.
3. Divide the meatballs into small portions (recipe makes
   30 meatballs), roll into balls with your hands, dust with
   flour and set aside.
4. Pour the tomato soup and tomato juice into a fairly large
   saucepan, add the water, and bring to the boil, then turn
   heat down to simmering temperature.
5. Drop the meatballs one by one into the tomato soup, spooning
   some liquid over each one to prevent them sticking together.
6. Cover the saucepan and allow the tomato soup to simmer
   gently until the meatballs are cooked, about 30 minutes.
   Turn the meatballs occasionally with a large spoon to
   prevent them sticking to the bottom of the pan.
7. Serve the meatballs in the gravy, garnished with parsley and
   accompanied by vegetables and rice or mashed potato.

Storage: Cover and refrigerate for up to three days.

Nutrition data per serve:
1377 kJ (329 cal), carbohydrate 38g, protein 24g, fat 8g, saturated
fat 2.9g, fibre 5g, sodium 573mg
GI rating: med

Meatloaf with spicy barbecue sauce

This meatloaf cooks in its own luscious, dark sauce.

Serves 4
Preparation/cooking time:
1 hour

500g (1lb) lean minced beef

3 slices of wholegrain bread, crumbed

1 onion, finely chopped

2 teaspoons curry powder

1 tablespoon chopped parsley

1 egg

½ cup skim or low-fat milk

½ cup water

½ cup tomato sauce

¼ cup Worcestershire sauce

2 tablespoons vinegar

1 teaspoon instant coffee

Juice of 1 lemon

1 tablespoon cornflour (cornstarch)

Method

1. Unless cooking in a microwave (see steps 5 and 10), preheat the oven to 180°C (350°F)
2. Combine minced beef, breadcrumbs, onion, curry powder, parsley and egg. Stir until mixture is well combined.
3. Add milk and continue mixing until mixture is smooth.
4. Shape meat mixture into a loaf and place in baking dish.
5. Bake in oven for 30 minutes, or microwave, covered, on medium for 20 minutes.
6. Remove from oven or microwave and drain off any fat.
7. While meatloaf is cooking, combine in a saucepan the water, tomato sauce, Worcestershire sauce, vinegar, coffee and lemon juice.
8. Bring slowly to boil, reduce heat and simmer for five minutes.
9. Pour sauce over meat and return to oven or microwave.
10. Bake for a further 20–30 minutes, basting frequently with sauce, or microwave on medium for a further 20 minutes.
11. Mix cornflour with 1 tablespoon of water to a smooth paste. Remove meatloaf to a serving plate and slice.
12. Add cornflour mixture to the sauce in the baking dish and bring back to the boil, stirring constantly until thickened.
13. Pour thickened sauce over the meatloaf. Serve hot with vegetables or cold with salad.

Storage: Keep in airtight container or cover with plastic film in refrigerator for up to two days. You can also freeze the meatloaf in an airtight container.

Nutrition data per serve:
1523 kJ (364 cal), carbohydrate 32g, protein 32g, fat 11g, saturated fat 4.2g, fibre 3g, sodium 809mg
GI rating: low

Beef stroganoff

Fusilli or spiral noodles make a good bed for this dish as the spirals hold the sauce.
Cook the pasta while you prepare the stroganoff.

Serves 4
Preparation/cooking time:
20 minutes

500g (1lb) porterhouse steak, trimmed

1 clove garlic, crushed or ½ teaspoon minced garlic

1 tablespoon Worcestershire sauce

1 medium onion

4 medium mushrooms

2 teaspoons cornflour (cornstarch)

1 cup skim or low-fat milk

1 tablespoon no-added-salt tomato paste

1 tablespoon oil

1 tablespoon chopped parsley

4 tablespoons natural yoghurt

Method

1. Slice beef across the grain, into thin strips about 7 centimetres (2½ inches) long and 1 centimetre (¼ inch) wide.
2. Place meat in a bowl and toss with garlic and Worcestershire sauce. Leave to marinate while you prepare remaining ingredients.
3. Roughly dice onion and slice mushrooms.
4. Blend cornflour with a little milk, then add remaining milk. Add the tomato paste and stir well, set aside.
5. Heat 2 teaspoons oil in a deep frying pan until very hot. Add meat and stir-fry for 3 minutes or until meat is browned all over. Remove from pan and set aside.
6. Heat remaining oil and add onions and mushrooms. Stir-fry for about 3 minutes or until vegetables are almost cooked.
7. Return meat to pan and stir in milk mixture. Stir gently until mixture boils and thickens.
8. Reduce heat and simmer for two minutes.
9. Serve on a bed of pasta, sprinkle with parsley and top each serve with 1 tablespoon yoghurt.

Nutrition data per serve:
1154 kJ (276 cal), carbohydrate 10g, protein 32g, fat 12g, saturated fat 3.8g, fibre 2g, sodium 177mg
GI rating: low

Indian lamb
in spinach sauce

This recipe is ideal served with Dry curry of potato, eggplant and pea (see page 146) and basmati rice or Spiced rice with peas (see page 135).

Serves 4
Preparation/cooking time:
1 hour 30 minutes

6 ripe tomatoes or 440g (15½oz) can tomatoes

1 tablespoon oil

2 cloves garlic, finely chopped

2 teaspoons finely chopped fresh ginger

2 fresh green or red chillies, finely chopped, or 1 teaspoon minced chillies

Salt to taste (optional)

500g (1lb) lean lamb, diced

1 teaspoon garam masala

500g (1lb) frozen spinach, thawed, or 2 bunches fresh spinach, finely chopped

Method

1. Blend tomatoes in a food processor.
2. Heat oil in saucepan, add garlic, ginger, chillies and salt. Cook, stirring, for two minutes.
3. Add lamb, mix well, cover and cook over low heat for 30–40 minutes or until lamb is tender. Stir occasionally.
4. Add tomatoes and cook for a further 10 minutes.
5. Add spices and simmer gently for 10 minutes.
6. Add spinach and simmer for a further four minutes.

Nutrition data per serve:
1267 kJ (303 cal), carbohydrate 6g, protein 33g, fat 14g, saturated fat 4.6g, fibre 9g, sodium 233mg
GI rating: low

Irish stew

Serves 4
Preparation/cooking time:
2 hours

600g (1¼lb) lamb leg chops,
trimmed of visible fat, bone left in,
meat cut into large pieces

2 cups Basic homemade chicken
stock (page 89)

¼ teaspoon white pepper

¼ teaspoon salt (optional)

1 teaspoon dried mixed herbs

2 medium onions,
roughly chopped

1 large carrot, peeled and sliced

8 small new potatoes (chats)

Optional—2 tablespoons plain
flour mixed with ¼ cup cooled
stock to thicken
—see Step 3.

2 tablespoons chopped parsley
to garnish

Method

1. In a large saucepan, combine the chops, stock, pepper, salt and herbs. Bring to the boil then reduce to a simmer with the lid on. Cook slowly 30 minutes.
2. Add the onions, carrot and potatoes and simmer for a further 30 minutes or until meat and vegetables are tender.
3. To thicken, lift meat and vegetables from the liquid and place in a serving dish, then add the flour mixed with cooled stock and bring the liquid to the boil, cooking until it has thickened, then pour over the meat and vegetables, garnishing with the chopped parsley.

Nutrition data per serve:
1293 kJ (309 cal), carbohydrate 18 g, protein 36g, fat 9g, saturated fat 4.4g, fibre 3g, sodium 111mg
GI rating: med

Seared kangaroo fillets

Kangaroo steaks can be used instead of fillets. This marinated meat is great cooked on the barbecue. Serve with mashed sweet potato flavoured with horseradish and green vegetables or serve sliced over Spinach and beetroot leaves salad (see page 211) with couscous.

Serves 4
Preparation/cooking time:
15 min
+ 10 min to marinate

1/3 cup red wine

Juice of half lemon

3 sprigs rosemary, roughly chopped

Black pepper

500g (1lb) kangaroo fillets

1 tablespoon oil

Method

1. Prepare the marinade. In a bowl, combine all the ingredients, except the kangaroo and oil.
2. Marinate kangaroo fillets for at least 10 minutes.
3. Heat oil in frying pan over high heat. Place kangaroo in pan, sear on 1 side for approximately 4 minutes and once it easily lifts from pan, turn over.
4. Cook for a further 4 minutes, Remove from heat, wrap in foil for 10 minutes to rest.
5. Slice and serve.

Storage: Kangaroo is best eaten freshly cooked but it can be covered and refrigerated for up to three days after cooking.

Nutrition data per serve:
747 kJ (179 cal), carbohydrate 0g, protein 27g, fat 6g, saturated fat 1.1g, fibre 0g, sodium 52mg

Kangaroo is gaining popularity in the Australian diet. It is presently a cheaper alternative to other red meats and is very low in fat but still rich in protein, iron and zinc.

The low-fat content of kangaroo meat means it is best cooked either quickly over high heat or slowly stewed to keep it moist. If searing or roasting, cook quickly, wrap it in foil and stand it for 10 minutes before slicing and serving.

Balanced eating: side dishes

Vegetables

Balanced eating: Add plenty of vegetables, salads and maybe some fruit, cooked or raw, as either the main part of a dish or as a side dish.

Vegetables add colour, flavour, texture and interest to meals, provide important vitamins, minerals and phytochemicals for health, and should be a part of all main meals. Unfortunately many people are unsure how to prepare them in a way that will tempt the whole family to eat them. If overcooked, many vegetables will lose colour and flavour and become mushy.

Vegetables are very versatile and can be served cooked or raw, as a separate course, as a major ingredient in or as an accompaniment to a dish. If your children are not keen on eating vegetables, try adding vegetables to soups and casseroles, grate into hamburgers or meat sauce or try our Sausage rolls (page 258), Pizzas (page 104), Dips (page 250) with raw vegetables, Stir fries (page 120) and other dishes and sauces that contain vegetables that are throughout this book. They may not accept all of these suggestions at first, do not force them but keep offering small serves.

Try mixing vegetables in different combinations, and experiment with adding fresh or dried herbs and seasonings. Nutmeg, curry powder, onion, chives, tomato, garlic, wine or a sprinkle of toasted sesame seeds or almonds provide a delicious flavour boost. Fruit can add another dimension to salads and savoury dishes.

Snow peas and asparagus

Cut 20 asparagus spears to about the length of the snow peas, discarding the woody ends. Plunge the asparagus into boiling water for two minutes until the asparagus spears are tender.

Add twenty snow peas, return to the boil and then drain. Make sure that the vegetables don't overcook.

Place them on a serving dish and sprinkle them with toasted sesame seeds or almond slivers.

This recipe can be varied by replacing the asparagus with whole green beans or celery strips that have been microwaved on high for two to three minutes.

Nutrition data per serve:
127 kJ (30 cal), carbohydrate 2g, protein 3g, fat 1g, saturated fat trace, fibre 2g, sodium 2mg

Pumpkin and mushrooms

Peel and seed 4 medium pieces of pumpkin and slice each into pieces about 1-centimetre (¼ inch) thick. Place them in a saucepan with 6 sliced mushrooms, 1 cup unsweetened tomato juice, 1 crushed clove garlic and ground black pepper.

Simmer gently for about 15 minutes until the vegetables are tender or, alternatively, place all the ingredients in a microwave dish, cover and microwave on high for eight minutes.

Nutrition data per serve:
213kJ (51cal), carbohydrate 1g, protein 3g, fat trace, saturated fat trace, fibre 2g, sodium 190mg

Zucchini creole

Peel and quarter 1 medium onion and cut ½ medium green capsicum into strips. Place in a saucepan with 2 tablespoons of water and cook for two minutes.

Add 4 quartered tomatoes, 4 small zucchini cut into 4, 12 pitted black olives and ½ teaspoon of chopped fresh basil (or ¼ teaspoon dried basil), cover and simmer gently for 10 minutes.

Nutrition data per serve:
124 kJ (30 cal), carbohydrate 5g, protein 1g, fat 0g, saturated fat 0g, fibre 1g, sodium 82mg

Orange-glazed carrots

Serves 4

Orange-glazed parsnips make a tasty alternative – replace 1 or both carrots with parsnip

Preparation/cooking time: 15 minutes

2 medium carrots, scrubbed and sliced

1 teaspoon grated orange rind

½ cup orange juice

2 teaspoons margarine

1 tablespoon chopped fresh chives or parsley

Method

1. Drop carrots into boiling water and cook until almost tender (about 5 minutes), or microwave, covered, with 2 tablespoons of water for three minutes until almost tender.
2. Drain and add orange rind, juice and margarine.
3. Bring to boil and cook for a further three minutes, or microwave, covered, on high for a further two minutes.
4. Lift out carrots and keep warm.
5. Return saucepan to heat and simmer orange sauce to allow it to reduce and thicken. Add the fresh herbs, pour the sauce over the carrots, and serve.

Nutrition data per serve:
156 kJ (37 cal), carbohydrate 4g, protein 0g, fat 2g, saturated fat 0.3g, fibre 1g, sodium 29mg

Sweet and sour red cabbage

Serves 4

Preparation/cooking time: 30 minutes

500g (1lb) red cabbage, shredded

1 onion, chopped

1 cooking apple, peeled, cored and chopped

1 clove garlic, crushed

1 tablespoon vinegar

1 teaspoon caraway seeds (optional)

Pepper to taste

3 tablespoons water

Method

1. Place cabbage, onion, apple, garlic, vinegar, caraway seeds (if using), pepper and water in a saucepan or microwave-proof bowl.
2. Cook over a low heat for five minutes, stirring frequently, or microwave on high for three minutes. Alternatively, spray a pan with oil, add the ingredients, and stir fry until cooked through (about 5 minutes).
3. Serve by arranging the cabbage on a hot serving dish, sprinkled with parsley.

Nutrition data per serve:
305 kJ (73 cal), carbohydrate 11g, protein 3g, fat trace, saturated fat trace, fibre 6g, sodium 24mg
GI rating: low

Lemon broccoli

Wash 1 large head of broccoli, removing the woody stem. Cut the broccoli into even florets and steam or boil them for four to six minutes until they are tender but still crisp. Drain the broccoli. Alternatively, microwave on high for 3–4 minutes.

Add the juice and rind of 1 lemon and 2 teaspoons toasted sesame seeds and toss together. Serve immediately.

Nutrition data per serve:
259kJ (62 cal), carbohydrate 1g, protein 3g, fat 1g, saturated fat trace, fibre 6g, sodium 33mg

Curried brussels sprouts with almonds

Most people say they won't eat sprouts, but once you serve them cooked this way, everyone will be back for more!

Serves 4
Preparation/cooking time:
10 minutes

20 brussels sprouts, with stems trimmed and bases slit

1 teaspoon margarine

2 tablespoons blanched, slivered almonds

2 teaspoons water

1 small onion, finely diced

1 teaspoon curry powder

Method

1. Drop the brussels sprouts into a saucepan containing 2 centimetres (¾ inches) of boiling water and boil rapidly for about five minutes, or until cooked, but still firm. Drain sprouts and set aside in a bowl.
2. Dry the saucepan and return to heat.
3. Melt margarine in saucepan, add almonds and toss until lightly brown. Remove from pan.
4. Add water, onion, and curry powder and stir until onions are lightly cooked.
5. Return sprouts and almonds to saucepan, toss to mix and serve.

Nutrition data per serve:
374 kJ (89 cal), carbohydrate 3.0g, protein 5g, fat 5g, saturated fat 0.4g, fibre 4g, sodium 36mg

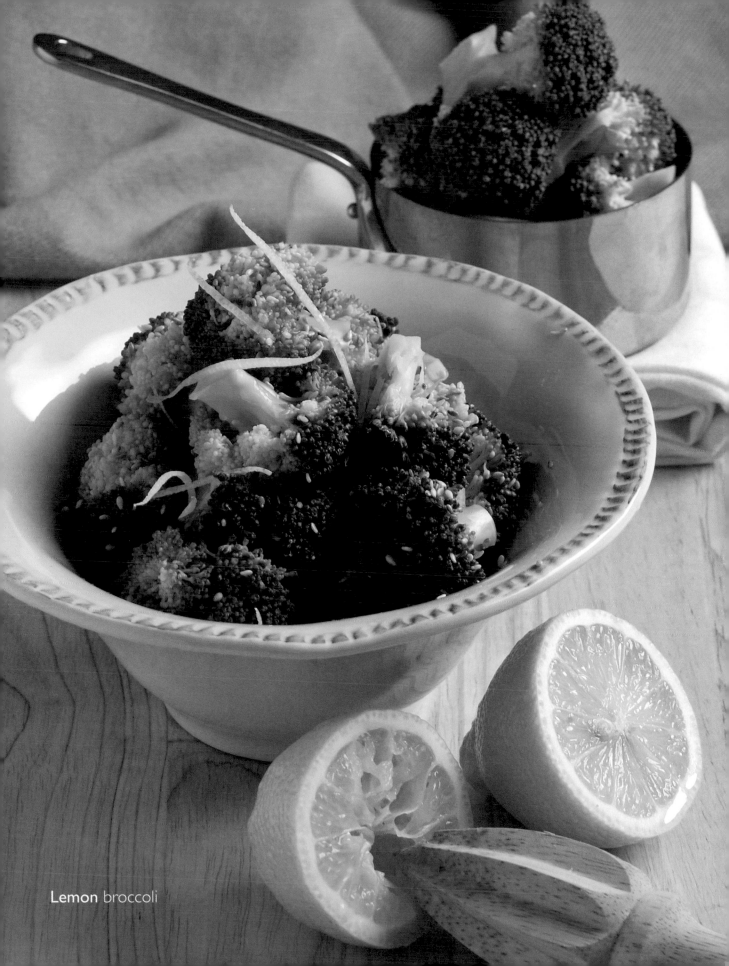

Lemon broccoli

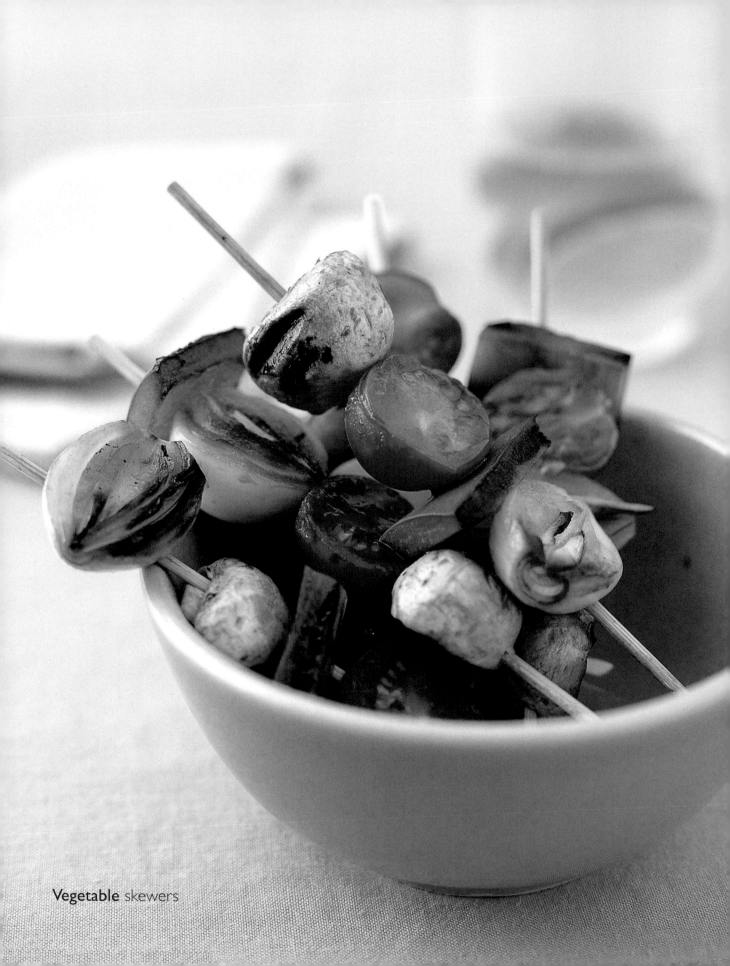

Vegetable skewers

Vegetable skewers

Serve these with rice or on a bed of cracked wheat and you have the basis of a delectable meal. Vegetable skewers are also really popular as part of a barbecue.

Serves 4
(8 skewers, 2 per serve)
Preparation/cooking time:
20 minutes

16 cherry tomatoes

16 pearl onions, peeled
(or small pieces of onion)

16 button mushrooms,
stalks trimmed

1 medium green capsicum cut
into 2cm squares

2 tablespoons lemon juice

2 teaspoons light soy sauce

Method

1. Thread vegetables evenly along eight 18-centimetre (7-inch) skewers, leaving about 2½ centimetres (1 inch) of skewer free at each end.
2. Mix lemon juice and soy sauce, and brush mixture over vegetables.
3. Grill for about five minutes on each side until vegetables are tender. During grilling, brush with lemon juice and soy sauce mixture at intervals to prevent drying.
4. Serve hot.

Nutrition data per serve:
244 kJ (58 cal), carbohydrate 8g, protein 3g, fat 0g, saturated fat 0g, fibre 3g, sodium 113mg
GI rating: low

Eggplant neapolitan

Serves 4
Preparation/cooking time:
1 hour

1 large or 2 small eggplants
(aubergine), peeled
and thinly sliced

4 large tomatoes, sliced

2 onions, sliced

½ teaspoon mixed dried herbs

Ground black pepper to taste

1 clove garlic, crushed

1 cup tomato juice or puree

Method

1. Preheat oven to 180°C (350°F)
2. Layer vegetables in casserole.
3. Sprinkle with herbs, pepper and garlic and pour over the tomato juice or puree.
4. Bake in oven, uncovered, for 45 minutes.

Nutrition data per serve:
277 kJ (66 cal), carbohydrate 9g, protein 4g, fat 0g, saturated fat 0g, fibre 5g, sodium 247mg
GI rating: low

Salads

Salads do not need to be complicated; some of the best ones are simple to prepare. Salads can add colour and texture to a meal and most can be prepared ahead of time.

Salads can be used alone as a meal or to accompany another dish. The recipes we give you here are planned as accompaniments but other salads are given in the Lunches and light meals section as well as Rice salad page 114, Curried pasta salad page 118 and Sweet potato salad page 151. The following suggestions are for four people:

Tossed salad

There are many different vegetables to toss in a salad. Just use your imagination. For instance, consider blanched green beans, zucchini, broccoli and cauliflower florets.
You can combine alfalfa sprouts, mushrooms, snow peas, sugar-snap peas, carrot and celery with the more traditional ingredients such as various kinds of lettuce, rocket, or beetroot greens, capsicum, cucumber and tomatoes. Avocado adds richness, as do olives.

1. Toss your choice of ingredients in ¼ cup low-fat or no fat Italian of French dressing. Always add dressing just before serving so vegetables remain crisp.

Asparagus and green bean salad

1. Trim eight spears of fresh asparagus and cut into 7-centimetre (2¾-inch) lengths.
2. Top, tail and halve 12 green beans. Boil, steam or microwave both vegetables until just tender, then drop into icy water to cool quickly. (This helps retain their crispness and colour.) Drain.
3. Tear a mignonette lettuce into pieces and line a salad bowl.
4. Combine the asparagus, beans and 16 cherry tomatoes and place in the salad bowl. Pour over ¼ cup low oil or no fat Italian dressing and sprinkle with 2 tablespoons of toasted sesame seeds.

Nutrition data per serve:
314 kJ (75 cal), carbohydrate 6g, protein 34g, fat 3g,
saturated fat 0.4g, fibre 3g, sodium 183mg
GI rating: low

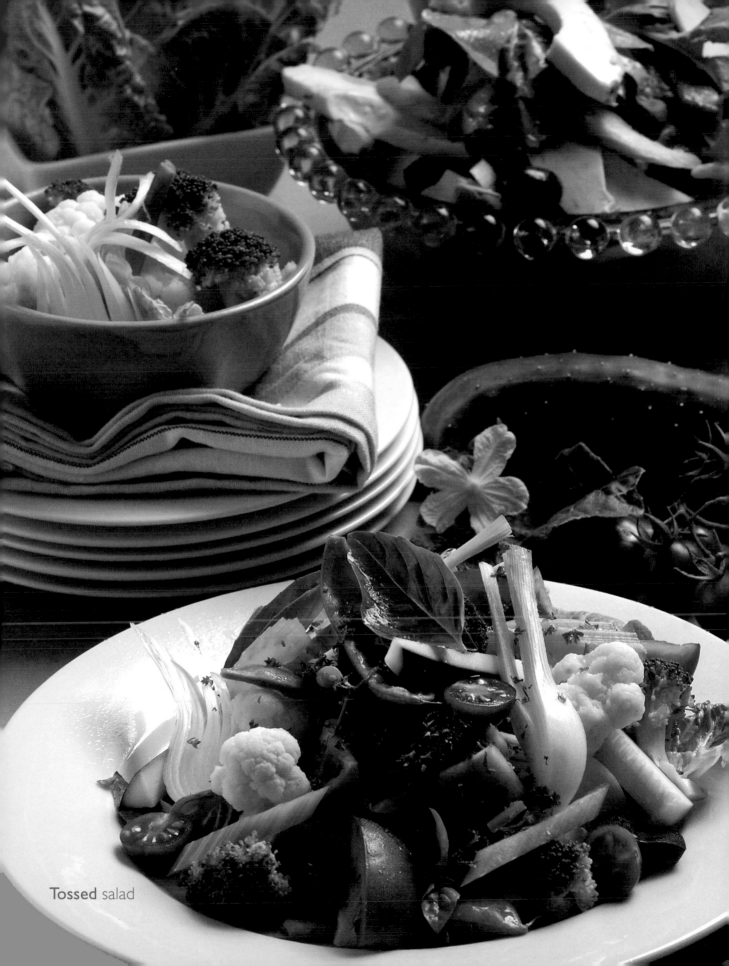

Tossed salad

Orange and cucumber salad

1. Peel and slice two oranges, removing all pith.
2. Slice half a cucumber and a small onion.
3. Break the onion into separate rings.
4. Mix orange, cucumber and onion and sprinkle with 1 tablespoon of chopped parsley.
5. Pour over one quantity of creamy orange dressing (see page 221).
6. Chill well before serving.

Nutrition data per serve:
237 kJ (57 cal), carbohydrate 9g, protein 3g, fat 0g,
saturated fat 0g, fibre 2g, sodium 33mg
GI rating: low

Avocado, spinach and orange salad

1. Wash a bunch of spinach, remove the stalks and tear the leaves into bite-size pieces. Place spinach in a bowl and add a sliced medium avocado, 12 pitted and quartered black olives, 1 Lebanese or ½ continental cucumber, sliced; and 1 orange, peeled and cut into segments.
2. Make a dressing of 1 tablespoon olive oil, 2 tablespoons lemon juice, a crushed clove of garlic, and 1 teaspoon mild sweet prepared mustard. Blend all together.
3. Pour it over the salad and toss lightly. Chill.

Nutrition data per serve:
910 kJ (218 cal), carbohydrate 7g, protein 4g, fat 19g,
saturated fat 3.6g, fibre 4g, sodium 117mg
GI rating: low

Tabbouleh

Serves 4
Preparation/cooking time:
1½ hours

½ cup burghul (cracked wheat)

2 large ripe tomatoes, skinned and finely chopped

1 small onion, finely chopped, or 4 spring onions, trimmed and finely sliced

1 cup chopped parsley

Freshly ground black pepper

1 tablespoon olive oil

3 tablespoons lemon juice

¼ cup finely chopped mint

Method

1. Place burghul in a deep bowl, cover with boiling water and allow to stand for 1 hour.
2. Drain well by squeezing in a clean muslin cloth or tea towel or in a sieve over a bowl, and return to bowl.
3. Add the tomatoes, onion, parsley, pepper, oil, lemon juice and mint.
4. Combine well and chill before serving.

Nutrition data per serve:
406 kJ (97 cal), carbohydrate 11g, protein 3 g, fat 3g, saturated fat 0.6g, fibre 4g, sodium 14 mg
GI rating: no GI available for burghul or cracked wheat but as it is made from the wholewheat grain this recipe is most probably low GI

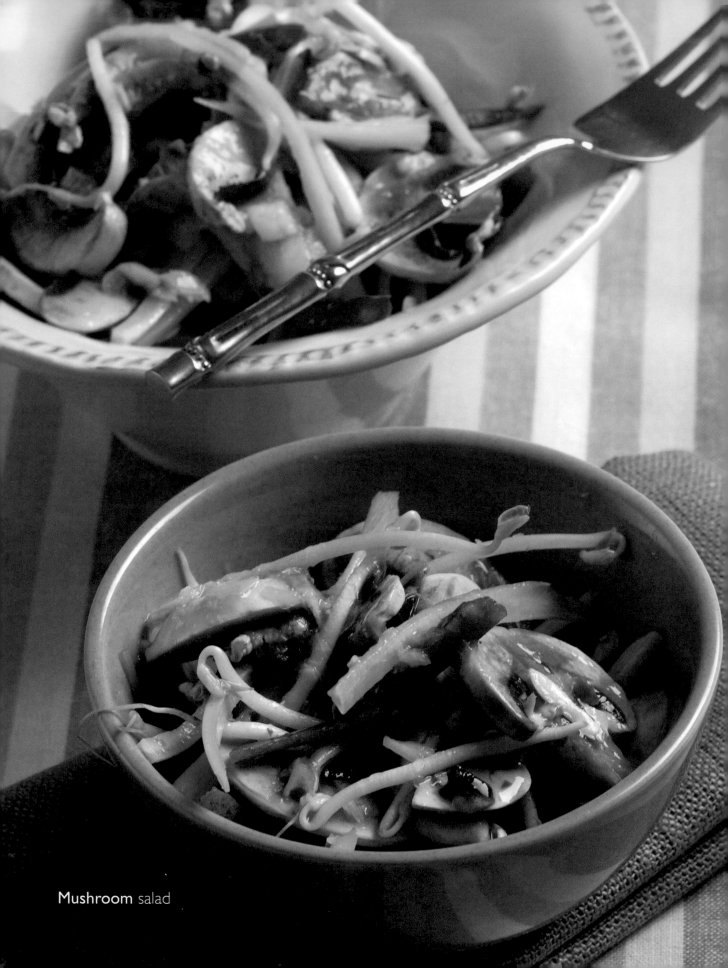

Mushroom salad

Mushroom salad

1. Slice 10 medium mushrooms into a bowl.
2. Add 1 cup beanshoots, ½ cup each celery and red capsicum, cut into matchsticks, and two chopped spring onions.
3. Toss with half a quantity of Orange and soy dressing (see page 221) and chill well.

Nutrition data per serve:
119 kJ (28 cal), carbohydrate 3g, protein 2g, fat 1g, saturated fat trace, fibre 2g, sodium 62mg

Spinach and beetroot leaves salad

A colour sensation—leaves can be purchased pre-mixed or if you grow beetroot in your garden, pick the beetroot young and use tender inside leaves.

Serves 4
Preparation/cooking time:
25 minutes

2 medium carrots, peeled

2 medium parsnips, peeled

4 baby or 2 medium beetroot, peeled

1 tablespoon oil

4 sprigs fresh rosemary

8 cups mixed baby spinach and baby beetroot leaves

1 quantity Orange and soy dressing page 221

Method

1. Preheat oven to 180°C (350°F)
2. Cut carrots, parsnips and beetroot to make about 12 pieces of each vegetable.
3. Toss in oil and place on oven tray.
4. Place in oven for 20 minutes or until cooked through and starting to brown.
5. While vegetables are cooking, wash salad leaves and place on a serving platter.
6. Sprinkle with dressing and top with hot vegetables.

Nutrition data per serve:
229 kJ (55 cal), carbohydrate 6g, protein 2g, fat 2g, saturated fat 0.8g, fibre 7g, sodium 181mg
GI rating: med

Hot Thai salad

This salad is really good as a salad to accompany
Thai fish cakes (see page 178), barbecued beef, chicken or seafood.

Serves 4
Preparation/cooking time:
10 minutes

2 medium carrots, peeled
and grated

1 bunch radish, grated

½ large continental cucumber,
grated or cut into thin strips

⅓ bunch coriander,
roughly chopped

1 quantity Hot Thai dressing
(see page 220)

¼ cup chopped roasted unsalted
peanuts

Method

1. Toss all vegetables and the coriander together in a large bowl.
2. Pour dressing over salad and top with the nuts.

Nutrition data per serve:
413 kJ (99 cal), carbohydrate 7g, protein 4g, fat 4g,
saturated fat 0.5g, fibre 2g, sodium 1307mg
GI rating: low

Spinach Valentino

Serves 4
Preparation/cooking time:
5 minutes

1 bunch spinach

4 mushrooms, sliced

2 spring onions, sliced

2 eggs, hard-boiled and sliced

1 quantity Orange and soy
dressing (see page 221)

Method

1. Wash spinach thoroughly, and shake gently to remove excess
   water. Remove the stalks and tear into bite-size pieces.
2. Combine spinach, mushrooms, spring onions and eggs and
   toss in dressing.
3. Chill before serving.

Nutrition data per serve:
312 kJ (75 cal), carbohydrate 2g, protein 6g, fat 4g,
saturated fat 0.9g, fibre 3g, sodium 145mg

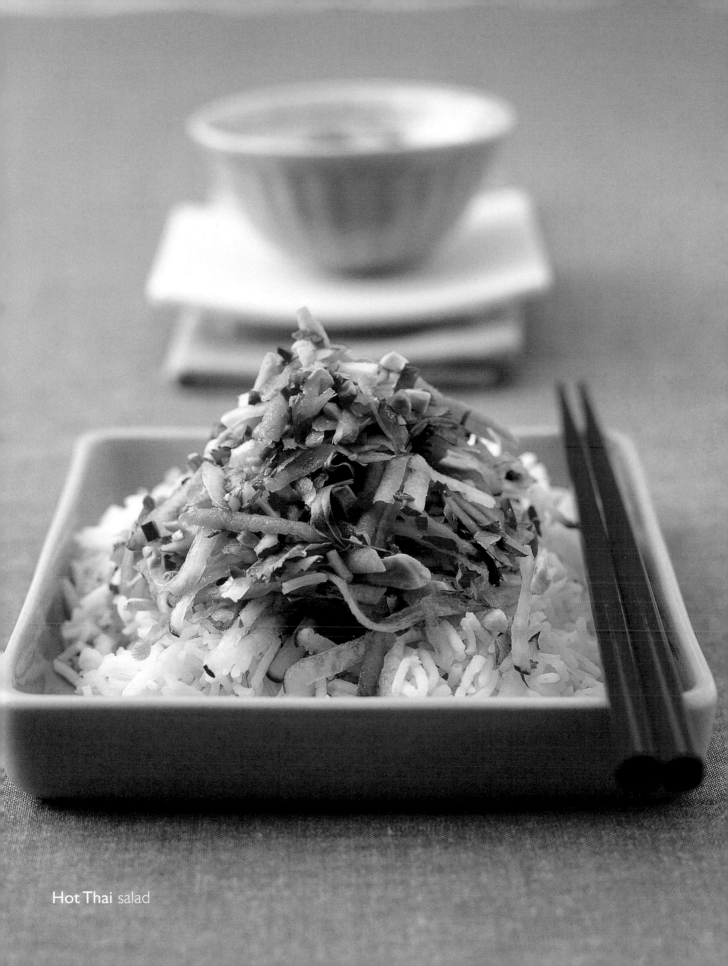

Hot Thai salad

Coleslaw

Once you have added the dressing, coleslaw should not be stored. However, you can prepare the vegetables in advance and store them in the refrigerator. Add the dressing just before serving.

Serves 4
Preparation/cooking time:
10 minutes

¼ medium cabbage,
finely shredded

1 small onion, grated or chopped
finely or 4 spring onions, trimmed
and sliced

1 small green or red capsicum,
chopped

1 stick celery, chopped

1 medium carrot, grated

Ground black pepper

½ cup low-fat coleslaw dressing

Method

1. Toss all prepared vegetables in a large bowl and chill until ready to serve.
2. Just before serving, pour the dressing over, toss all together, and serve.

Variations

Add 1 green apple, peeled, cored, and cut into small dice, or ½ cup pineapple cut into small dice.

Make the dressing more piquant by adding 1 teaspoon prepared mild mustard, 1 teaspoon sugar, and 1 tablespoon vinegar or lemon juice.

Storage: Cover and refrigerate for no more than a day.

Nutrition data per serve:
167 kJ (40 cal), carbohydrate 4g, protein 2g, fat trace, saturated fat trace, fibre 4g, sodium 197mg

Sauces, dressings and marinades

Sauces and dressings add flavour, interest and improve the appearance of many dishes. Traditionally many are high in fat, so here we show you how they can tantalise your taste buds without the fat.

Balanced eating: flavour

White sauce

Serves 4
Makes 2 cups
Preparation/cooking time:
15 minutes

1 tablespoon margarine

2 tablespoons plain flour

2 cups low-fat milk

½ teaspoon nutmeg

Pepper and salt (optional) to taste

Method

1. Melt margarine in a small saucepan

2. While still over the heat, add the flour and stir with a spoon until both are well combined.

3. Add ½ cup milk, reduce heat, and cook, stirring constantly, while the flour mixture absorbs the milk, then stir briskly to make sure there are no lumps.

4. Add a further ½ cup milk and repeat step 3

5. Add the nutmeg, pepper and salt, then the remainder of the milk and stir while the mixture comes to the boil, then simmer, stirring, until you have a smooth sauce. Check flavour and adjust to your taste.

Nutrition data per serve:
477 kJ (114 cal), carbohydrate 11g, protein 6g, fat 5g, saturated fat 1.6g, fibre trace, sodium 100mg
GI rating: low

Cheese sauce

Serves 4
Preparation/cooking time:
20 minutes

Makes 2¼ cups

1 quantity White Sauce (as above)

½ cup grated low-fat tasty or block cheese

pinch paprika

Method

1. Make white sauce. When the sauce is finished, add the cheese and paprika, stir until the cheese has melted.

Nutrition data per serve:
602 kJ (144 cal), carbohydrate 11g, protein 11g, fat 6g, saturated fat 2.3g, fibre trace, sodium 198mg
GI rating: low

Satay (peanut) sauce

Serves 4
Makes 2 cups
Preparation/cooking time:
15 minutes

1 small onion, grated

1 clove garlic, crushed

½ –1 teaspoon minced or finely chopped fresh chillies

½ cup crunchy low-salt peanut butter

6 teaspoons (1½ tablespoons) light soy sauce

1 tablespoon lemon juice

1 tablespoon sugar

2 teaspoons sweet chilli sauce

1 teaspoon grated or minced fresh ginger

½ cup water

Method

1. Spray a frying pan with spray oil. Add onion and garlic and cook gently until soft.
2. Add chilli, stir in and cook for one minute over medium heat.
3. Add peanut butter and stir. Add soy sauce, lemon juice, sugar, sweet chilli sauce, ginger and water and mix well. Bring mixture to boil, stirring constantly. Reduce heat and simmer gently for one minute. Check flavour and adjust to your taste.

Nutrition data per total quantity:
567 kJ (136 cal), carbohydrate 4g, protein 6g, fat 10g, saturated fat 107g, fibre 2g, sodium 185mg

Sweet and sour sauce

Serves 4
Preparation/cooking time:
15 minutes

440g (15½oz) can pineapple
pieces in natural juice

1 tablespoon white vinegar

2 teaspoons brown sugar

1 teaspoon light soy sauce

2 tablespoons tomato sauce

1 teaspoon grated or minced
fresh ginger

1 tablespoon cornflour
(cornstarch)

Method

1. Drain the juice from the pineapple and set both juice and fruit aside

2. Combine the vinegar, sugar, soy sauce, tomato sauce and ginger in a small saucepan.

3. Add 3 tablespoons pineapple juice to the cornstarch, mix together well to remove all lumps. Add this mixture to the ingredients in the saucepan, then pour the remainder of the juice in and stir over low heat until the mixture thickens.

4. Add the pineapple, stir again while it returns to the boil.

5. Serve with fish, chicken, or pork dishes—see stir-fry information on pages 120–129.

Nutrition data per serve:
334 kJ (80 cal), carbohydrate 18g, protein 1g, fat trace, saturated fat 0g, fibre 2g, sodium 151mg
GI rating: med

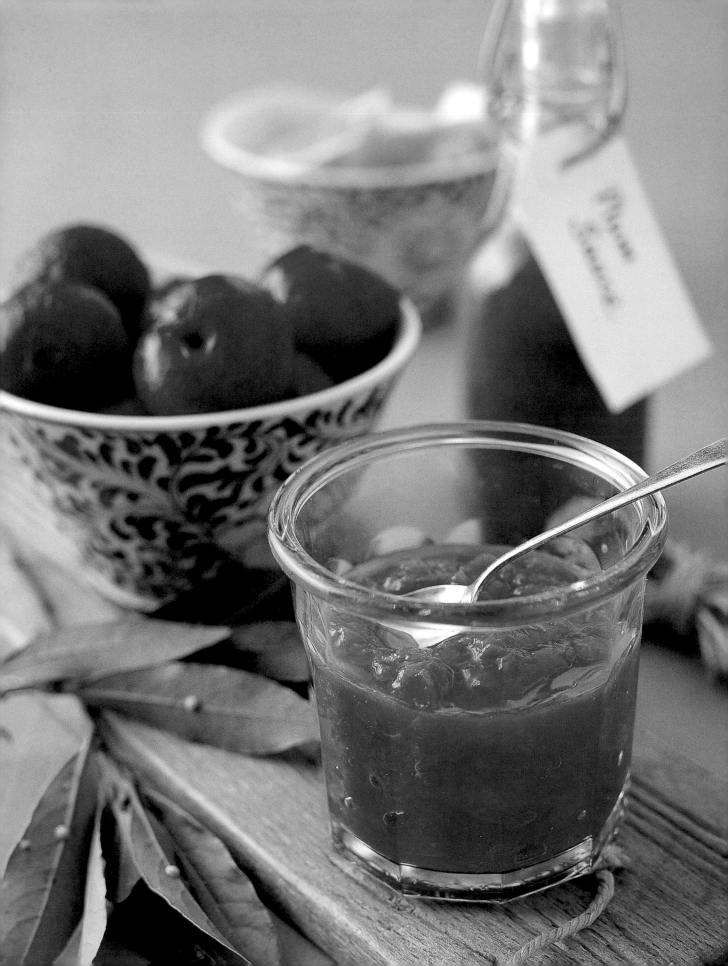

Plum sauce

Makes 1 litre
(1 tablespoon per serve)
Preparation/cooking time:
1 hour 30 minutes

2 onions, chopped

1 cup water

1kg (2¼lb) fresh plums, stoned

1 cup fresh orange juice

2 teaspoons grated or minced
fresh ginger

½ teaspoon whole cloves

¼ teaspoon peppercorns

Pinch of thyme

Pinch of oregano

1 bay leaf

Method

1. Lightly sauté onions in 2–3 tablespoons of the water, for two minutes.
2. Add the rest of the ingredients and cook over low heat, stirring regularly.
3. Simmer, with the lid off, for at least one hour until the mixture thickens.
4. Pour into clean warmed jars, allow to cool and then seal.

Storage: Keep in sealed jars in the refrigerator.

Nutrition data per total quantity:
2252 kJ (538 cal), carbohydrate 101g, protein 10g, fat 1g, saturated fat 0g, fibre 24g, sodium 59mg

Hot Thai dressing

Makes ¾ cup (1 tablespoon per serve)
Preparation/cooking time: 5 minutes

2 tablespoons light soy sauce

2 tablespoons fish sauce

2 tablespoons mirin (rice wine)

3 tablespoons lemon juice

2 small hot red chillies, seeded and finely chopped
or ½–1 teaspoon minced chillies

1 teaspoon grated or minced fresh ginger

2 teaspoons sugar

Method

1. Place soy sauce, fish sauce, mirin, lemon juice, chillies, ginger and sugar into a screw top jar and shake well.
2. Use as required.

Nutrition data per tablespoon:
63 kJ (16 cal), carbohydrate 2g, protein 1g, fat 0g, saturated fat 0g, fibre 0g, sodium 571mg

Curry dressing

Makes ½ cup (Serves 4)
Preparation/cooking time: 5 minutes

½ cup low-fat natural yoghurt

2 teaspoons hot curry powder or paste

2 tablespoons chopped parsley

½ teaspoon minced garlic (optional)

Method

1. Mix all ingredients and adjust flavourings to taste.
2. Chill and use same day.

Nutrition data per serve:
88 kJ (21 cal), carbohydrate 2g, protein 2g, fat trace, saturated fat 0g, fibre trace, sodium 24mg

Orange and soy dressing

Makes ¼ cup (Serves 4)
Preparation/cooking time:
5 minutes

¼ cup unsweetened orange juice

2 teaspoons light soy sauce

1 clove garlic, crushed,
OR ½–1 teaspoon minced garlic

1 teaspoon oil
(preferably sesame oil)

Method

1. Combine all ingredients in a screw top jar.
2. Chill and shake well before use.

Storage: Cover and refrigerate for up to two days.

Nutrition data per serve:
73 kJ (17 cal), carbohydrate 1g, protein trace, fat 1g,
saturated fat 0g, fibre trace, sodium 93mg

Creamy orange dressing

Makes ¾ cup (Serves 4)
Preparation/cooking time:
5 minutes

¼ cup unsweetened orange juice

2 teaspoons grated orange rind

1 tablespoon finely chopped
parsley

2 teaspoons finely chopped chives

½ cup low-fat natural yoghurt

Method

1. Combine all ingredients and chill.

Storage: Cover and refrigerate for up to two days.

Nutrition data per serve:
100 kJ (24 cal), carbohydrate 3g, protein 2g, fat trace,
saturated fat 0g, fibre 0g, sodium 24mg

Tomato relish

**Makes 3.5 litres
(1 tablespoon per serve)
Preparation/cooking time:
1 hour 30 minutes**

3 large onions

2½ kg (5½lb) chopped,
ripe tomatoes

5 large granny smith apples,
cored and chopped (skins left on)

3 cups vinegar

500g (1lb) sultanas

3 cloves of garlic, crushed

1 cup fresh orange juice

1 teaspoon mixed spice

4 whole cloves

1 teaspoon chilli powder

Method

1. Place all the ingredients in a large saucepan and bring to the boil. Turn the heat to low and simmer for one hour, stirring frequently. Remove from heat.
2. Pour hot water into clean jars to warm them. Pour water away.
3. Fill jars with hot chutney. Allow them to cool, then seal the jars and store.

Storage: Keep in sealed jars. Once opened, store in refrigerator.

Nutrition data per total quantity:
11971 kJ, (2862 cal), carbohydrate 588g, protein 53g, fat 7g, saturated fat trace, fibre 82g, sodium 460mg

Other sauces

In this book, sauces or dressings are matched with recipes they complement although you might like to try them with a different dish.

For instance:

- Check the Pasta section for several useful sauces page 137
- Cherry sauce with beef fillet page 264
- Strawberry and peppercorn sauce with chicken page 268

Quick and easy marinades

The following recipes can be used to marinate barbecued or grilled meats. Quantities are for 500g (1lb) of meat and will serve four. Stir ingredients, and use to brush meat as it grills.

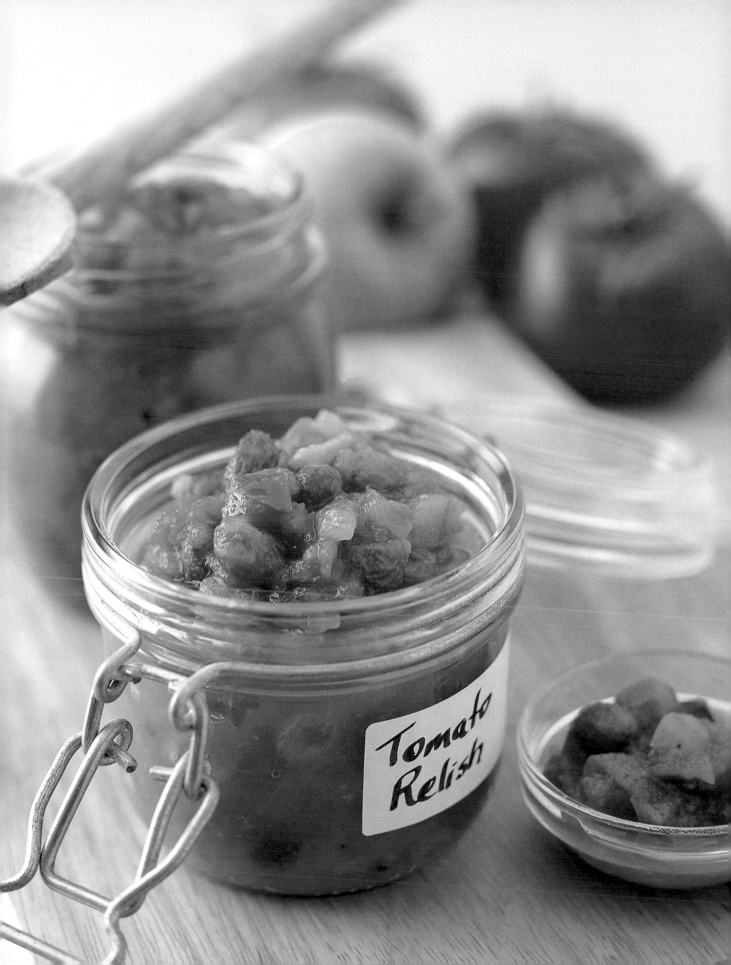

Tomato Relish

Red wine marinade

Combine ½ cup dry red wine, 1 tablespoon no-salt tomato paste, 1 tablespoon Worcestershire (or soy, or teriyaki) sauce, 2 tablespoons finely chopped parsley, 1 clove crushed garlic, ground black pepper to taste and ¼ teaspoon finely chopped oregano or basil (optional).

To 'rev it up', add: ¼ cup sweet chilli sauce and/or, 1–2 cloves crushed garlic or 1 teaspoon minced garlic.

Nutrition data per serve:
128 kJ (31 cal), carbohydrate 2g, protein trace, fat trace, saturated fat 0g, fibre trace, sodium 71mg

Singapore sizzler marinade

Combine 2 tablespoons sweet chilli sauce, 2 tablespoons light soy or teriyaki sauce, 1 tablespoon lemon or lime juice, 2 teaspoons sugar and 1 teaspoon finely chopped or minced fresh ginger.

Nutrition data per serve:
157 kJ (36 cal), carbohydrate 8g, protein 1g, fat 0g, saturated fat 0g, fibre 0g, sodium 442mg

Greek lamb

Particularly good for lamb is a combination of ¼ cup no-added-salt tomato paste, ¼ cup water, 2 teaspoons Worcestershire sauce, 2 teaspoons chopped fresh or ½ teaspoon dried rosemary, 2 cloves crushed garlic (or 1 teaspoon minced), dash of Tabasco sauce and four chopped spring onions.

Nutrition data per serve:
85 kJ (20 cal), carbohydrate 3g, protein 1g, fat trace, saturated fat 0g, fibre 1g, sodium 42mg

Barbecue marinade

Combine ¼ cup white wine vinegar, 2 tablespoons sugar, ½ cup no-added-salt tomato sauce, 2 tablespoons Worcestershire sauce, and 1 teaspoon prepared mild mustard. Marinate meat for at least 1 hour. Marinade can be used to brush over meat as it is cooking

Nutrition data per serve:
328 kJ (78 cal), carbohydrate 19g, protein 1g, fat trace, saturated fat 0g, fibre 1g, sodium 149mg

Desserts and sweet treats

Fruit and dairy foods make a good basis for many desserts

Dessert can be a nutritious component of a meal. Fruits and dairy foods make a good basis to many desserts, are mainly low GI foods and add vitamins and minerals as well as carbohydrates.

Here you will also find some baked items like cakes. We have put these into this section to encourage you to use them as occasional sweet treats rather than on a daily basis.

This section gives you some easy and tasty ideas that are suitable for the whole family and for friends.

Creamy rice

Serves 6
Preparation/cooking time:
1 hour

1 cup arborio rice

1½ cups water

2½ cups skim or low-fat milk

½ teaspoon ground nutmeg

1 teaspoon vanilla essence

1 tablespoon sugar or equivalent artificial sweetener

Method

1. Wash rice and place in saucepan, cover with the water, and simmer over very low heat until water is absorbed.
2. Add 1 cup milk. Simmer again until absorbed. Stir occasionally to prevent rice sticking to the bottom of the saucepan.
3. Add the remaining 1½ cups milk and cook again until the milk is absorbed.
4. Stir in nutmeg, vanilla and sugar or sweetener to taste.
5. Serve warm with sliced stewed or fresh fruit.

Storage: Cover and refrigerate for up to three days.

Nutrition data per serve:
694 kJ (166 cal), carbohydrate 35g, protein 6g, fat trace, saturated fat 0g, fibre 0g, sodium 49mg
GI rating: low

Custard sauce

Serves 4
Preparation/cooking time:
15 minutes

3 level tablespoons custard powder

2 cups skim milk

1 teaspoon vanilla

1 tablespoon sugar, or the equivalent of Equal™, Splenda™ or other artificial sweetener

Method

1. Blend custard powder and a small quantity of the milk to make a smooth paste.
2. Place remaining milk in saucepan and bring to boil.
3. Gradually stir in custard paste. Return to heat and continue stirring until mixture thickens. Add vanilla and sugar or artificial sweetener.
4. Simmer for one minute, stirring constantly.

Variation: Add 1 teaspoon of finely grated orange rind to milk before heating.

You can serve this sauce hot or cold.

Nutrition data per serve:
373 kJ (89 cal), carbohydrate 17g, protein 5g, fat trace, saturated fat trace, fibre 0g, sodium 58mg
GI rating: low

Brandy sauce

Serves 4
Preparation/cooking time:
20 minutes

1 quantity of custard sauce (see recipe above)

1 egg, separated

2 tablespoons brandy

Method

1. Beat egg yolk and add to custard sauce with the custard powder paste (Step 1).
2. Whip egg white until peaks form.
3. When custard has cooked, fold egg white through custard and add brandy.
4. Serve immediately.

Nutrition data per serve:
533 kJ (127 cal), carbohydrate 18g, protein 6g, fat 1g, saturated fat 0.5g, fibre 0g, sodium 75mg
GI rating: low

Pastry

Pastries are traditionally high in fat but here we show you how to make a low-fat fruit strudel using Filo pastry. Filo is almost fat free and adapts well to a variety of uses. We use a cooking spray to separate the layers and maintain crispness. Filo pastry can be readily purchased in the supermarket, either fresh or frozen, although the fresh version, if available, is easier to use.

Apple strudel

All the pleasure of the traditional strudel, but with a fraction of the fat.

Serves 6
Preparation/cooking time:
45 minutes

5 sheets filo pastry

Cooking spray

4 apples, peeled and very finely sliced or 1 x 400g (14oz) can pie apple

4 tablespoons sultanas

2 tablespoons chopped pecans or walnuts

1 teaspoon cinnamon

¼ teaspoon ground cloves

1 tablespoon brown sugar

¼ cup crushed shredded wheatmeal biscuits

Nutrition data per serve:
830 kJ (198 cal), carbohydrate 34g, protein 3g, fat 6g, saturated fat 0.9g, fibre 4g, sodium 119mg
GI rating: low

Method

1. Preheat oven to 200°C (400°F)
2. Cook the apples if using fresh apple, allow to cool.
3. Combine the apple with the sultanas, nuts, spices, sugar, and wheatmeal biscuits.
4. Spread one sheet of pastry on a kitchen bench, and spray lightly with cooking spray.
5. Place another layer of pastry on top. Again spray with oil.
6. Repeat for remaining sheets of pastry.
7. Spread the fruit mixture over the pastry, leaving a 2-centimetre (¾-inch) space around the edges.
8. Spray a baking tray with non-stick baking spray, or cover with baking paper.
9. Carefully roll up the pastry. Place on the baking tray, loose edge down.
10. Spray the strudel top with oil. Bake in oven for 25–30 minutes or until golden brown and heated through.
11. Serve warm, cut into thick slices, with warm custard.

This recipe will freeze. For variety, substitute apple with apricots or other fruit.

Fruit crumble

You can replace the apples in this recipe with peaches, apricots or plums or with two apples and half a cup of cooked rhubarb. If you have a favourite combination, you can use it in this recipe, too.

*If the fruit mixture is not sweet enough for your taste,
add a little sugar or your preferred sweetener.*

Serves 6
Preparation/cooking time:
1 hour

4 large eating apples, peeled, cored and sliced

2 tablespoons water

½ teaspoon ground cinnamon

¼ teaspoon ground cloves

⅓ cup sultanas
or chopped dried apricots

Topping:
1 cup quick cooking oats

¼ cup desiccated coconut

¼ cup slivered almonds

½ teaspoon cinnamon

1 tablespoon sugar

1 tablespoon margarine

Method

1. Preheat the oven to 180°C (350°F)
2. Place apple into a saucepan, add water, spices and dried fruit.
3. Simmer gently for approximately 10 minutes until apple is tender, or microwave, covered, on high for six minutes.
4. Lightly grease a small casserole and spoon in apple mixture.
5. Mix oats, coconut, almonds, cinnamon, and sugar. Rub the margarine into the mixture until it crumbles. Spread over the top of the fruit.
6. Bake in oven for 30 minutes or until topping becomes golden. Serve hot or cold with custard or fruit yoghurt.

Storage: Cover and refrigerate for up to four days.

Nutrition data per serve:
960 kJ (230 cal), carbohydrate 34g, protein 3g, fat 9g, saturated fat 2.6g, fibre 5g, sodium 22mg
GI rating: low

Baked custard

This family favourite can be served hot or cold.

**Preparation/cooking time:
1 hour 10 minutes**

4 eggs

3 tablespoons sugar or equivalent
artificial sweetener

2 cups skim or low-fat milk

1 teaspoon vanilla essence

Sprinkle of ground nutmeg
(optional)

Method

1. Preheat the oven to 180°C (350°F)
2. Lightly beat the eggs in a bowl.
3. Gradually add the milk to the egg mixture, stirring constantly. Stir in the vanilla essence and sugar or sweetener.
4. Pour mixture into a deep pie or soufflé dish or four single-serve oven proof dishes. Sprinkle with nutmeg.
5. Stand the baking dish(es) in a large deep baking dish. Carefully pour enough water into the large baking dish to reach two-thirds up the outside of the custard dish(es).
6. Bake in oven for 30–35 minutes if you are using individual dishes, 40 minutes if you are using one big dish. The custard should be lightly browned on top and just set in the centre.

Nutrition data per serve:
687 kJ (164 cal), carbohydrate 19g, protein 11g, fat 5g, saturated fat 1.7, fibre 0g, sodium 124mg
GI rating: low

Fruity baked rice pudding

Serves 6
Preparation/cooking time:
2 hours

3½ cups skim or low-fat milk

½ cup arborio rice

Artificial sweetener to taste or
1 tablespoon sugar

1 teaspoon vanilla essence

⅓ cup sultanas or raisins

½ cup dried peaches
or apricots, chopped

2 teaspoons margarine

Ground nutmeg or cinnamon,
for garnish

Method

1. Preheat the oven to 180°C (350°F)
2. Combine 2½ cups milk, the rice, sugar (if using) and dried fruit in a baking dish.
3. Cover and bake in oven for 30 minutes.
4. Remove from oven and stir, adding a further ½ cup milk, stirring in well.
5. Leave uncovered and return to oven. Cook for another 30 minutes.
6. Then add the final ½ cup milk and the margarine, stir and return to the oven and cook a further 30 minutes. A skin will have formed on top of the rice.
7. Stir in artificial sweetener (if using).
8. Serve hot or cold, garnished with ground nutmeg or cinnamon.

Storage: Cover and refrigerate for up to three days.

Nutrition data per serve:
721 kJ (172 cal), carbohydrate 32g, protein 7g, fat 1g,
saturated fat trace, fibre 2g, sodium 83mg
GI rating: low

Bread and butter pudding

Serves 4
Preparation/cooking time:
1 hour

3 eggs

2 cups skim or low-fat milk

1 teaspoon vanilla essence

2 tablespoons sugar

3 slices wholegrain
or sourdough bread

2 teaspoons margarine

2 tablespoons sultanas

1 teaspoon ground nutmeg

Method

1. Preheat the oven to 180°C (350°F)
2. Place eggs in bowl and beat.
3. Add milk, vanilla essence, and sugar and mix well together.
4. Spread bread with margarine and cut each slice into four squares.
5. Place cut bread in the base of a deep baking dish, margarine side up.
6. Sprinkle sultanas and nutmeg evenly over the bread, then pour the custard mixture carefully over the top.
7. Place the dish in a larger baking dish, and carefully pour water into the larger baking dish to reach two-thirds up the outside of the custard dish.
8. Bake in oven for 45–60 minutes or until just set.
9. Serve hot or cold with fresh or stewed fruit.

Nutrition data per serve:
1041 kJ (249 cal), carbohydrate 35g, protein 13g, fat 7g, saturated fat 1.8, fibre 2g, sodium 299mg
GI rating: low

Thick pancakes or pikelets

On page 148 we show you how to make thin pancakes or crepes. These ones contain a little sugar and are thick which makes them suitable for stacking and topping with a sweet mixture. Pikelets make a good snack or addition to a lunch box.

Serves 6 (1 thick pancakes or 2 pikelets per serve)
Preparation/cooking time:
20 minutes + 1 hour standing time for batter

¾ cup white self-raising flour
¾ cup wholemeal self-raising flour
1 tablespoon sugar (optional)
1 egg, lightly beaten
1 tablespoon margarine, melted
1¼ cup skim or low-fat milk
Spray oil

Method

1. Place flours and sugar into a bowl and make a well in the centre.
2. Slowly add the beaten egg, melted margarine and then the milk, stirring continually to draw the ingredients together and prevent lumps forming.
3. Mixture should be the consistency of thickened cream. If you prefer, use a food processor or blender and simply add all the ingredients at once and process until smooth.
4. Leave to stand in a cool place for at least an hour. If the mixture has thickened too much, add more milk, a little at a time, to the consistency of thickened cream.
5. Lightly spray a non-stick frying pan with oil and heat until very hot, but not smoking.
6. Drop spoonfuls of mixture into pan allowing room for each pancake or pikelet to spread.
7. When mixture begins to bubble, turn over with a spatula or egg slice.
8. Let pancakes/pikelets cook until light brown on each side and lift onto a clean cloth. Keep covered with a damp tea-towel until you need them.

Nutrition data per serve:
769 kJ (184 cal), carbohydrate 29g, protein 7g, fat 4g, saturated fat 0.9g, fibre 3g, sodium 170mg
GI rating: low

Berry and cheese pancakes

Serves 6
Preparation/cooking time:
5 minutes

2 cups mixed berries, washed
and hulled

1 teaspoon water

1 tablespoon sugar

6 Thick pancakes
(see page opposite), warmed

6 tablespoons smooth ricotta
cheese

Method

1. Poach berries in water with the sugar for approximately
   three minutes until soft and the juice starts to run.
2. Divide fruit evenly between pancakes and top each with
   1 tablespoon ricotta cheese.
3. Serve hot.

Nutrition data per serve:
951 kJ (227 cal), carbohydrate 30g, protein 10g, fat 6g, saturated
fat 2.4g, fibre 4g, sodium 215mg
GI rating: low

Look for other sweet pancake recipes

Breakfast: Apple and sultana pancakes page 76

Meals for special occasions: Flambéed crepes and Crepes suzette page 171

Baked apples with orange and strawberry sauce

Serves 4
Preparation/cooking time: 1 hour

4 apples
(e.g. granny smith or pink lady)

½ teaspoon ground cinnamon

1 cup orange juice

1 punnet (250g/9oz) strawberries

1 tablespoon sugar or equivalent artificial sweetener

2 tablespoons slivered almonds or chopped pecans

Orange slices

Method

1. Preheat the oven to 180°C (350°F)
2. Peel and core apples. When peeling, leave some peel on, to create a horizontal striped effect.
3. Place in a small baking dish. Sprinkle with cinnamon, then pour on the orange juice.
4. Bake, covered, in oven for 30–35 minutes, or microwave on high for six to eight minutes, until the apples are tender but still retain their shape. Baste occasionally to prevent drying out.
5. While apples are cooking, wash, hull and puree strawberries.
6. Add sugar or sweetener to the puree.
7. When apples are cooked, lift gently onto individual serving dishes.
8. Reduce cooking liquid by boiling if necessary, and pour onto strawberry puree. Mix and pour over apples.
9. Decorate with slivered nuts and orange slices.
10. Serve warm or chilled.

Storage: Cover and refrigerate for up to two days.

Nutrition data per serve:
796 kJ (190 cal), carbohydrate 31g, protein 4g, fat 4g, saturated fat 0.3g, fibre 6g, sodium 10mg
GI rating: low

Ginger pears

Serves 4 (1 pear per serve)
Preparation/cooking time:
1 hour

4 medium pears, peeled
and quartered

285ml (9½fl oz) bottle low-joule
(low-calorie) dry ginger ale

Juice of 1 lemon

½ teaspoon minced fresh ginger

¼ cup orange juice concentrate

6 cloves

Ground cinnamon, for garnish

Method

1. Place pears in a saucepan. Add dry ginger ale, lemon juice, ginger, orange juice concentrate, and cloves.
2. Cover and simmer until pears are tender, turning and basting the pears so they cook and colour evenly. Alternatively, microwave, covered, on high for four to six minutes until tender.
3. Lift pears onto serving dish.
4. Simmer juice until slightly reduced.
5. Pour over pears. Sprinkle with cinnamon.
6. Serve hot or chilled.

Storage: Cover and refrigerate for up to four days.

Nutrition data per serve:
493 kJ (118 cal), carbohydrate 27g, protein 1g, fat 0g,
saturated fat 0g, fibre 3g, sodium 5mg
GI rating: low

Spiced oranges

This is an ideal dessert after a long, hot summer's day.

Serves 6
Preparation/cooking time:
15 minutes

2 cups red wine

1 cup unsweetened orange juice

1 tablespoon sugar or equivalent
artificial sweetener

½ teaspoon ground cinnamon
or 2 cinnamon sticks

6 oranges

Method

1. Place wine, orange juice and cinnamon in a saucepan and bring to the boil.
2. Boil hard for two minutes, then remove from heat, or microwave on high for two to three minutes. Add the sugar or sweetener.
3. Peel oranges, removing all pith, slice horizontally and arrange in a glass serving bowl.
4. Pour wine mixture over oranges.
5. Chill well before serving.

Storage: Cover and refrigerate for up to four days.

Nutrition data per serve:
566 kJ (135 cal), carbohydrate 16g, protein 2g, fat 0g, saturated fat 0g, fibre 3g, sodium 14mg
GI rating: low

Desserts and sweet treats

If you have a microwave, use it to help make dessert preparation quick and easy, for example baked apples in strawberry sauce, ginger pears, spiced oranges. It can also save on dirty dishes. For example fruit cooks very well in the microwave, and making custard sauce in the microwave is very much quicker and easier than using a saucepan.

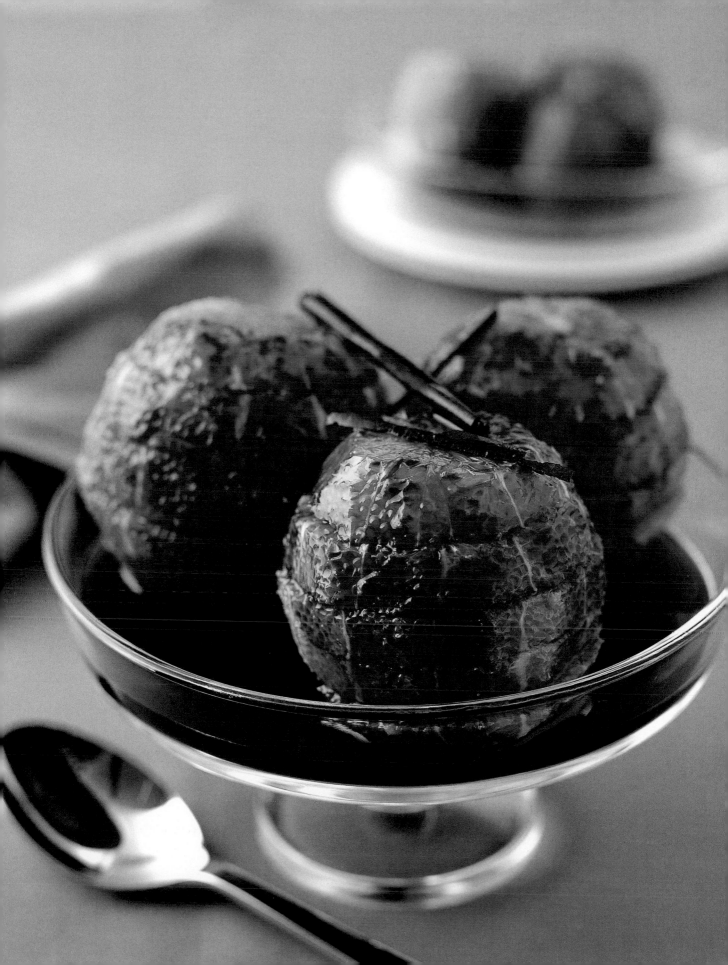

Lemon delicious

Serves 4
Preparation/cooking time:
1 hour

3 eggs

5 tablespoons fresh lemon juice

Rind of 1 lemon, grated

3 teaspoons melted margarine

3 tablespoons wholemeal plain flour

1½ cups low-fat milk

1 tablespoon sugar or equivalent artificial sweetener

Method

1. Preheat oven to 160°C (320°F)
2. Separate eggs. Beat egg whites until stiff peaks form.
3. Beat yolks with the remaining ingredients until smooth.
4. Gradually fold the egg whites into mixture.
5. Spoon evenly into four dishes.
6. Place in a larger baking dish. Carefully pour water into the larger baking dish until it reaches two-thirds up the outside of the individual baking dishes.
7. Bake in oven for approximately 20 minutes or until set and lightly browned.
8. Cool slightly in the water-filled dish to prevent shrinking.

Storage: Cover and refrigerate for one day only.

Nutrition data per serve:
654 kJ (156 cal), carbohydrate 12g, protein 11g, fat 7g, saturated fat 1.8g, fibre 1g, sodium 127mg
GI rating: low

A hint for fruit juice: to get more juice from citrus fruit, first microwave the whole fruit on high for one to two minutes. Stand for 30 seconds, then squeeze out the juice.

Very berry yoghurt

*This very wicked dessert is for yoghurt lovers only! It does use higher fat yoghurt,
but as the serve size is small it is fine for an occasional very special treat—and it makes
a wonderful dessert for dinner with friends—they will be so impressed and it is SO EASY!*

Serves 6
Preparation/cooking time:
10 minutes + draining time
for yoghurt

500g (17fl oz) Greek style yoghurt

2 cups mixed berries—frozen
or fresh (do not thaw if frozen)

2 tablespoons sugar

Method

1. Spoon all the yoghurt into a clean tea towel or 3-4 layers
   of cheesecloth. Gather the ends together, tie firmly at the
   top so the yoghurt is completely enclosed, and hang the
   bag of yoghurt over a bowl so the liquid that drains away
   is not touching the bottom of the bag. You can do this in a
   cool place (a laundry trough is good if the room is cool), or
   hang the yoghurt bag over a long-handled spoon suspended
   over a bowl and placed in the bottom of the refrigerator.
   This takes about 12 hours, so overnight is a good time to do
   it. The yoghurt, when ready, is a fairly firm mixture.

   Alternative 1: Place it in a mixing bowl, add berries and
   sugar and fold together so the fruit is well distributed
   through the yoghurt but some of the white yoghurt remains.
   Serve in small bowls.

   Alternative 2: place the berries and sugar in a small
   saucepan or bowl. Heat 3–4 minutes in the saucepan or
   1–2 minutes in the microwave—just long enough to warm
   the berries and release the juice. Stir well to blend the
   flavours and make a sauce.

2. Spoon some of the yoghurt into serving dishes, then spoon
   sauce over and serve.

Nutrition data per serve:
571 kJ (137 cal), carbohydrate 15g, protein 5g, fat 6g,
saturated fat 3.8g, fibre 1g, sodium 56mg
GI rating: low

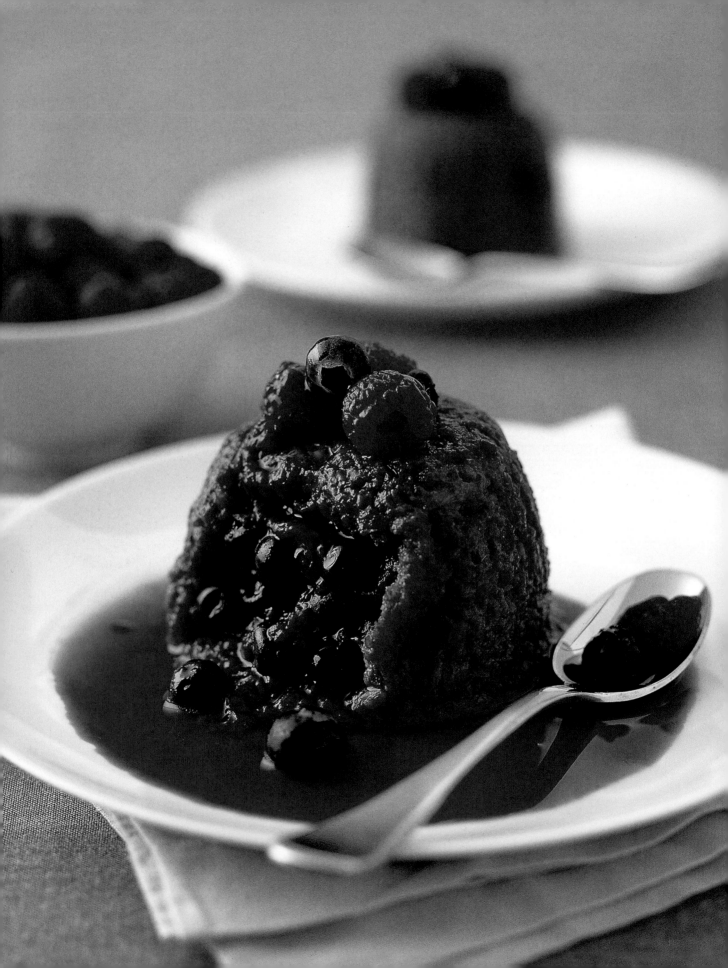

Summer pudding

Serves 6
Preparation/cooking time:
20 minutes + overnight
refrigeration

14 slices wholegrain or low GI
white bread, crusts removed

6 cups mixed fresh berries
(strawberries, raspberries,
blueberries, loganberries)

2 tablespoons caster sugar

Extra berries, for garnish

Method

1. Cut crusts off bread and discard them.
2. Cut six round bases and tops out of bread. Set tops aside. Place a base in six individual soufflé dishes. Use the remaining bread to line the sides of the dishes. Do this carefully, making sure that there are no gaps.
3. Wash and hull berries. Chop strawberries.
4. Place berries and sugar in saucepan, and heat gently until liquid runs from berries.
5. Fill soufflé dishes, packing fruit down firmly, and pour over the juice, distributing this evenly over the six moulds. Cover each with one of the reserved tops.
6. Place a weight on top and refrigerate overnight.
7. Turn onto serving dishes. Garnish with extra berries.

Nutrition data per serve:
876 kJ (209 cal), carbohydrate 33g, protein 7g, fat 2g, saturated fat trace, fibre 10g, sodium 210mg
GI rating: low

Flours

There are times when the texture or flavour of the dish is better made with wholemeal or stone ground flours. At other times a mixture of wholemeal and white flours or white flour only is better. We have used a mixture in our recipes.

Using wholemeal flour products gives a heavier or denser texture than white flour, and requires more liquid during cooking. We allow for this in our recipes.

Using the oven

Always preheat your oven so it is at the correct temperature when you are ready to bake.

Carrot cake

Makes twenty slices (1 slice per serve)
Preparation/cooking time: 1 hour

1 cup wholemeal self-raising flour

1 cup self raising flour

½ teaspoon bicarbonate of soda

2 teaspoons ground cinnamon

½ teaspoon ground nutmeg

1 teaspoon mixed spice

2 cups grated carrot

½ cup shredded coconut

½ cup chopped walnuts

½ cup sultanas

2 eggs

½ cup caster sugar

1 cup skim or low-fat milk

Method

1. Preheat oven to 200°C (400°F)
2. Grease and lightly flour a cake tin.
3. Sift flour, soda and spices. Return bran to flour mixture.
4. Add carrot, coconut, nuts and sultanas.
5. Beat eggs until fluffy and add sugar. Beat again and add milk.
6. Fold into dry ingredients. Stir until well mixed and pour batter into a prepared 20-centimetre (8-inch) cake tin.
7. Bake in oven until cooked through (approximately 50 minutes).
8. Turn out and cool on a cake rack.

Variation: Use pecans instead of walnuts.

Storage: Keeps in an airtight container for up to four days.

Nutrition data per slice:
548 kJ (131 cal), carbohydrate 19g, protein 3g, fat 4g, saturated fat 1.5g, fibre 2g, sodium 132mg
GI rating: med

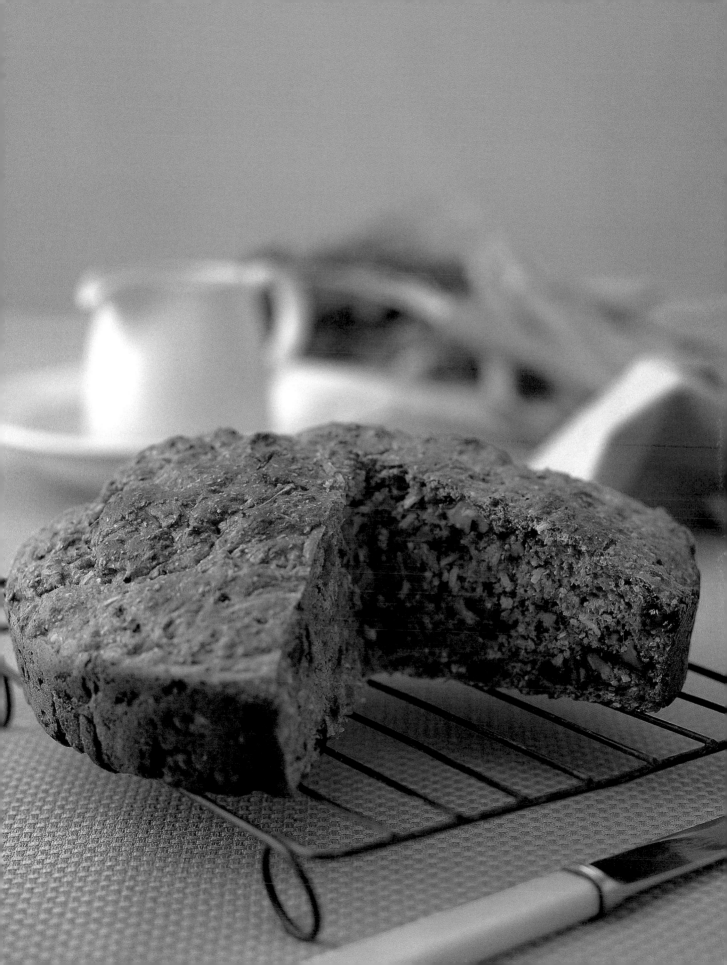

Apricot and walnut loaf

**Makes 12 slices
(1 slice per serve)
Preparation/cooking time:
1 hour 10 minutes**

½ cup boiling water

1 cup chopped dried apricots

¾ cup wholemeal self-raising flour

¾ cup self raising flour

1 teaspoon mixed spice

1 teaspoon ground cinnamon

2 tablespoons salt-reduced margarine

¼ cup sugar

½ cup chopped walnuts

1 egg, beaten

1 cup skim or low-fat milk

Method

1. Preheat the oven to 190°C (375°F)
2. Pour boiling water over apricots and let stand for 30 minutes.
3. Mix flours and spices in bowl.
4. Rub in margarine until mixture resembles breadcrumbs.
5. Add sugar, apricots, soaking water and walnuts to dry mixture and mix lightly.
6. Stir in egg and milk.
7. Place in lightly greased loaf tin.
8. Bake in oven for 30 minutes, then lower heat to 180°C (350°F). and bake for a further 20–25 minutes or until cooked.
9. Leave in tin for 10 minutes before turning out to cool.

Variation: Replace apricots and walnuts with any dried fruit of your choice.

Nutrition data per slice:
717 kJ (171 cal), carbohydrate 22g, protein 5g, fat 7g, saturated fat 0.8g, fibre 3g, sodium 151mg
GI rating: low

Baked yoghurt slice

Serves 8
Preparation/cooking time:
1 hour

10 shredded wheatmeal biscuits

2–3 tablespoons unsweetened apple juice, for base

1 cup low-fat fruit yoghurt

1 cup low-fat ricotta cheese

Juice and grated rind of 1 lemon

2 tablespoons unsweetened apple juice, for filling

2 egg whites

½ cup sultanas

Method

1. Preheat the oven to 180°C (350°F)
2. Grind the biscuits in food processor or blender or crush well with rolling pin.
3. Add apple juice to biscuit crumbs to make a spreadable mixture.
4. Line tart tin with aluminium foil.
5. Press the biscuit crumb mixture into lined tart tin.
6. Blend yoghurt, ricotta cheese, lemon juice and rind and apple juice in food processor or blender.
7. Beat egg whites until stiff. Fold through the blended cheese mixture with the sultanas. Pour into biscuit base.
8. Bake in oven for approximately 30 minutes until firm.
9. Cool and cut into slices.

Variation: Use different flavoured yoghurt.

Storage: Cover with plastic film and refrigerate for up to two days.

Nutrition data per slice:
723 kJ (173 cal), carbohydrate 23g, protein 7g, fat 5g, saturated fat 3g, fibre 1g, sodium 157mg.
GI rating: low

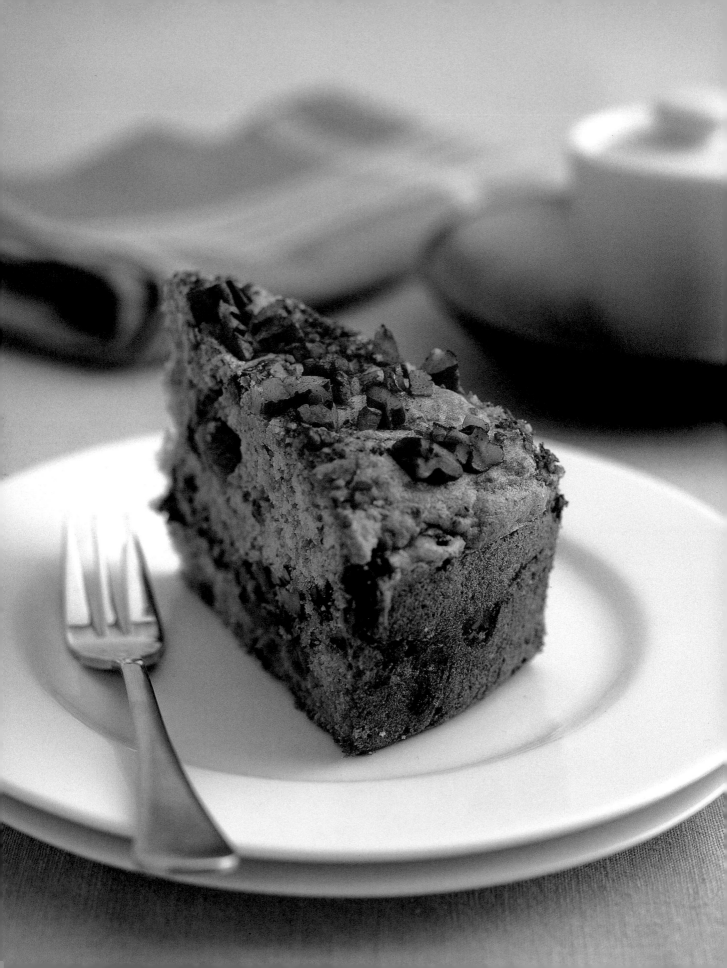

Wholemeal apple
and nut streusel cake

**Makes twenty slices
(1 slice per serve)
Preparation/cooking time:
1 hour 15 minutes**

120g (4¼oz) reduced salt
margarine

½ cup sugar

150g (5¼oz) low-fat ricotta cheese

1 teaspoon vanilla essence

3 eggs

1 cup white self-raising flour

1 cup wholemeal plain flour

1 teaspoon bicarbonate of soda

2 teaspoon cinnamon

1 cup skim or low-fat milk

1 apple, peeled and grated

1 cup sultanas

¾ cup chopped pecans or walnuts

1 tablespoon caster sugar

Method

1. Preheat the oven to 180°C (350°F)
2. Lightly grease and line the base of a 20-centimetre (8-inch) cake tin.
3. Cream margarine and sugar, then beat in ricotta and vanilla essence until the mixture is smooth.
4. Add eggs one at a time and beat in.
5. Mix flours, 1 teaspoon cinnamon and soda and fold into mixture with milk.
6. Add apple and sultanas and mix.
7. Combine the chopped nuts, remaining 1 teaspoon cinnamon, and 1 tablespoon sugar.
8. Spread half the cake mixture into the cake tin. Sprinkle over half the nut mixture. Spread with remaining cake mixture and sprinkle with remaining nut mixture.
9. Bake in oven for one hour or until cooked.
10. Cool slightly before turning out.

Storage: Cover and refrigerate for up to four days.

Nutrition data per slice:
804 kJ (192 cal), carbohydrate 22g, protein 4g, fat 9g,
saturated fat 1.7g, fibre 2g, sodium 175mg
GI rating: med

Nibbles and party foods

Here we give you some ideas for parties and pre-dinner nibbles. Some are higher in fat than others (see nutrition data for recipe) so these ones are better saved for special occasions.

Dips and dippers

As well as the recipes we provide here, there are several good low-fat biscuits and biscuit alternatives and dips that you can buy at your local supermarket. Read the product label (see page 62) and look for the GI or Tick symbols (see pages 64–65).

Pita crisps

You can use either pita bread or mountain bread for this. If using pitas, split in half.
Cut or tear into shapes. Place on oven tray and spray lightly with oil.
You can leave them unseasoned or sprinkle with any of the following:
- Lemon pepper
- Paprika
- Cajun spice
- Dried mixed herbs
- Curry powder
- Pepper and salt

Bake in a moderate oven 160°C (325°F) for 10–15 minutes or until lightly browned and crisp. Allow to cool. They can be stored in an airtight container for later use.

Alternatively, place a paper towel on microwave oven turntable, place pieces of the bread on the paper, and microwave on high for 1-2 minutes, depending on the power of your oven.

Prawn crackers

1 packet dry prawn crackers (available in the Asian food section of supermarket)

Place a paper towel on the turntable of microwave oven. Place 8–10 crackers on the paper, spreading out so they don't touch. Cook on high 35–45 seconds, depending on the power of the oven. The crackers will puff up and become light and crisp. Take care not to over-cook as they will burn. Experiment with a few to start, but remember that the more you cook at the same time, the longer it will take.

Poppadums

1 packet plain or flavoured poppadums (available in the Asian food section of the supermarket).

Place a paper towel on the microwave turntable. Place dry poppadums on the paper (not touching) and cook on high for 20–30 seconds (depending on the power of the microwave oven). They will puff up and increase in size. Be careful not to cook for too long as they will burn.

Alternatively, before placing the poppadums on the paper towel, spray with a little spray oil.

Potato wedges

1. Preheat oven to 200°C–220°C (400–425°F)
2. Cut two medium potatoes, skin on, into wedges and steam or microwave until partly cooked.
3. Place in a large mixing bowl and add herbs or seasonings as desired (see ideas for pita crisps). Mix well until the potatoes are well mixed with the seasonings.
4. Spray with a little spray oil, spread out on baking paper on a baking sheet and bake until golden brown and crispy—about 30–45 minutes. Turn once during cooking period.
5. Serve with tomato-based salsa or a low-fat dip.

Nutrition data per total quantity:
941 kJ (225 cal), carbohydrate 40g, protein 7, fat 2g, saturated fat 0.3g, fibre 6g, sodium 9mg
GI rating: high

Vegetables dippers

Vegetables that work well as 'dippers' include:

- Carrot, celery, cucumber, capsicum sticks or strips
- Snow peas
- Broccoli or cauliflower florets
- Baby mushrooms
- Spring onions

Dips

Good commercial dips include:

- Low-fat pre-prepared dips—check the fat content and aim for fat content of less than 10% fat i.e., less than 10g per 100g dip
- Fruit or mango chutney—these work well with poppadums, potato wedges
- Tomato-based salsa

Homemade dips

These dips also make excellent toppings for jacket potatoes, and some work well in other recipes.

French onion

1 tablespoon per serve
Preparation/cooking time:
10 mins

125g (4½oz) low-fat
(80% fat reduced) cream cheese

125g (4½oz) smooth ricotta cheese

½ packet French onion soup mix

Method

1. Place cream cheese in a mixing bowl and allow to soften.
2. Add the ricotta cheese and the soup powder and mix well together.
3. You can add chopped parsley or chives if you wish.

Variation: Replace onion soup mix with dried mushroom soup mix.

Nutrition data per tablespoon:
133 kJ (32 cal), carbohydrate 1g, protein 2g, fat 2g, saturated fat 0.6g, fibre 0g, sodium 26mg

Tsatziki

This also makes a tasty topping for grilled lamb, lamb or beef kebabs, or spoon onto fish for a tangy garnish.

1 tablespoon per serve
Preparation/cooking time:
10 mins

½ continental cucumber

200g (7fl oz) natural low-fat yoghurt

½–1 teaspoon minced garlic

Pepper and salt (optional) to taste

2 teaspoons chopped fresh parsley or mint

1 tablespoon chopped spring onion

Method

1. Grate cucumber (with skin on), place in a sieve or colander and drain until most of the liquid has been removed—use a spoon or your hand to push as much fluid out as possible.
2. Place in a mixing bowl, add all other ingredients and stir to combine. Refrigerate until ready to serve.

Nutrition data per tablespoon:
53 kJ (13 cal), carbohydrate 1g, protein 1g, fat trace, saturated fat trace, fibre 0g, sodium 12mg

Hummus

1 tablespoon per serve
Preparation/cooking time:
15 mins

1 x 400g (14oz) can chickpeas

¼ cup lemon juice

1–2 teaspoons minced garlic

2 tablespoons tahini paste

Paprika (optional)

1 tablespoon chopped fresh parsley

Method

1. Drain and rinse the chickpeas.
2. Grind in a food processor with the garlic, lemon juice and tahini until smooth and creamy. You may need to add a little water if the mixture looks stiff, but add carefully to avoid making the mixture too runny.
3. Add the seasonings, mix briefly again, spoon into serving bowl and refrigerate until ready to serve.

Note: Tahini is a paste of ground or crushed sesame seeds.

Nutrition data per tablespoon:
240 kJ (57 cal), carbohydrate 5g, protein 3g, fat 3g, saturated fat 0.4g, fibre 2g, sodium 86mg

Sweet and sour cheese dip

1 tablespoon per serve
Preparation/cooking time:
4 minutes + time taken
to make sauce

½ quantity Sweet and sour sauce,
(see page 217)

250g (8¾oz) low-fat
(80% fat reduced) cream cheese

Method

1. Place sweet and sour sauce in saucepan and gently heat.
2. Place cheese on a small shallow serving bowl, tip warm sauce over and serve immediately with pita crisps or low-fat dry biscuits.

Nutrition data per tablespoon:
149 kJ (36 cal), carbohydrate 2g, protein 1g, fat 2g, saturated fat 1.5g, fibre trace, sodium 64mg

Salmon dip

This is a great way to increase your fish intake!

1 tablespoon per serve
Preparation/cooking time:
15 mins

125g (4½oz) low-fat (80% fat
reduced) cream cheese

½ cup low-fat yoghurt or smooth
ricotta cheese

210g (7½oz) can pink
or red salmon

½–1 teaspoon curry powder

1–2 tablespoons lemon juice
(according to taste)

1 tablespoon chopped fresh
chives or parsley

Method

1. Drain the liquid from the salmon, remove any black skin and the bones.
2. Soften the cream cheese, add the yoghurt or ricotta, then the salmon and the seasonings.
3. Mix well together and adjust flavour to your taste.
4. Chill until ready to serve.

Nutrition data per tablespoon:
175 kJ (42 cal), carbohydrate 1g, protein 4g, fat 2g, saturated fat 0.4g, fibre 0g, sodium 21mg

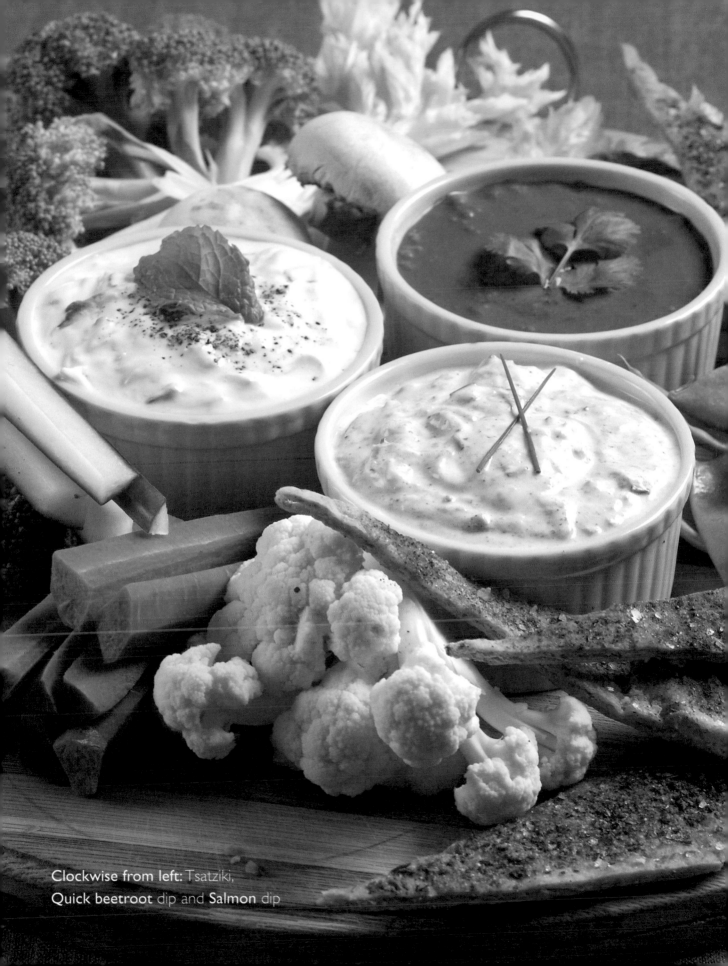

Clockwise from left: Tsatziki,
Quick beetroot dip and **Salmon** dip

Spicy Mexican dip

1 tablespoon per serve
This dip also works very well as a filling for tacos.
Preparation/cooking time: 10 mins

400g (14oz) cooked or canned and drained red kidney beans

½ red (Spanish) onion, chopped

¼ cup water

½ x 300g (10½oz) jar tomato-based salsa or ½ packet taco seasoning

Optional: 1 tomato, finely chopped

Method

1. Drain and rinse the kidney beans, place beans in food processor.
2. Add the onion, water, and salsa and process until smooth.
3. Spoon into a serving bowl and add the chopped tomato if using, folding this in lightly.

Nutrition data per tablespoon:
85 kJ (20 cal), carbohydrate 3g, protein 2g, fat trace, saturated fat 0g, fibre 2g, sodium 2mg

Quick beetroot dip

1 tablespoon per serve
Preparation/cooking time: 10 mins

225g (8oz) can beetroot, drained

¼ cup low-fat natural yoghurt or smooth ricotta cheese

1 teaspoon ground coriander

1 teaspoon ground cumin

2 tablespoons tahini paste

1 tablespoon lemon juice

Method

1. Add all ingredients to food processor and blend until smooth and creamy.
2. Check flavour, adjust to your taste, and refrigerate until ready to serve.

Nutrition data per tablespoon:
140 kJ (34 cal), carbohydrate 2g, protein 1g, fat 2g, saturated fat trace, fibre 1g, sodium 63mg

Vegetable samosas

Serves 6
(2 samosas per person)
Preparation/cooking time:
1 hour

2 potatoes, peeled and cut into small dice

1 tablespoon oil

1 teaspoon mustard seeds

1 onion, peeled and finely chopped

½–1 tablespoon mild curry paste

½ teaspoon ground garam masala (optional)

1 teaspoon minced fresh ginger

¾ cup frozen peas

2 tablespoons chopped fresh coriander

1 tablespoon lemon juice

12 sheets filo pastry

Spray oil

Method

1. Preheat oven to 180°C (350°F)
2. Cook the potatoes until tender, drain.
3. Add the oil to a frying pan, heat then add mustard seeds and cook, stirring until they start to pop, then add the onion and cook until soft.
4. Add the curry paste, garam masala, peas and ginger, and cook for 2–3 minutes.
5. Add the cooked potato, combine all ingredients, including the fresh coriander and lemon juice, and allow to cool a little.
6. Check and adjust flavour—you may wish to add a little salt and/or pepper.
7. Place 1 sheet pastry on a bench, spray with oil, cover with a second sheet, then repeat with a third. Cut into 5 strips along the wide side of the pastry.
8. Place a small amount of filling on one end of each strip of pastry, then fold over cornerwise until all the pastry is used and you have a triangle shape.
9. Place samosas on a baking sheet with the last pastry fold to the bottom, and spray lightly with spray oil. Bake in oven for approximately 15 minutes or until brown.
10. Serve with mango chutney or plum sauce.

Nutrition data per serve
713 kJ (170 cal), carbohydrate 24g, protein 5g, fat 5g, saturated fat 0.7g, fibre 3g, sodium 266mg
GI rating: high

Nibbles and party foods

Pumpernickel savouries

Many different combinations can be used to top rounds or squares of pumpernickel to make interesting and tasty savouries. Try these ideas:

- baby prawns or shrimps and avocado
- smoked salmon slices or rolls garnished with capers
- sliced hard-boiled egg topped with black caviar and tiny sprigs of parsley
- circles or squares of lean ham with asparagus tips
- low-fat cottage or low-fat ricotta cheese topped with strawberry halves, slices of peach or nectarine, or chopped dried figs or dates.

Nachos

Serves 6 as an appetiser
Preparation/cooking time:
20–30 minutes

1 large round wholegrain or plain pita bread

¾ cup (100g) (3½oz) grated low-fat mozzarella cheese

Salt (optional) and pepper, freshly ground, to taste

½ large or 1 small ripe avocado

2 tablespoons onion, shallot or spring onion, finely chopped

2 tablespoons lemon juice

4–5 drops tabasco sauce

4 tablespoons low-fat natural yoghurt

½ cup commercial tomato-based salsa

Method

1. Preheat oven to 180°C (350°F)
2. Split the pita bread and cut into shapes as for pita crisps (see page 248).
3. Place the dried crisps in a shallow baking dish and sprinkle the cheese over the crisps. Add pepper, and salt if desired. Place the crisps in oven until the cheese melts and the crisps are hot
4. While the crisps are cooking, mash the avocado with the onion, lemon juice, tabasco sauce, pepper and salt, mixing well so the mixture is fairly smooth. Place in a serving bowl.
5. Spoon the yoghurt into a serving bowl.
6. Spoon the salsa into a serving bowl.
7. Serve the dish of crisps with the avocado mixture, yoghurt and the salsa.

Nutrition data per serve:
629 kJ (150 cal), carbohydrate 11g, protein 8g, fat 8g, saturated fat 2.9g, fibre 2g, sodium 288mg
GI rating: low

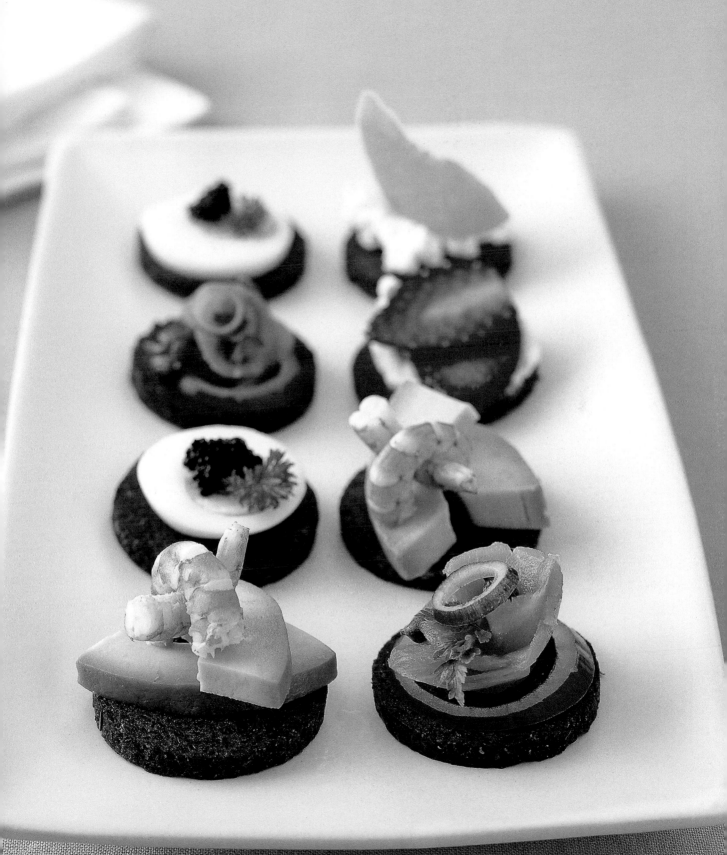

Pumpernickel savouries

Sausage rolls

Makes 32
Preparation/cooking time:
45 minutes

1 quantity rissole mixture

½ cup frozen peas

1 small sweet potato, peeled
and grated

¼ cup dry breadcrumbs extra

3 tablespoons tomato sauce

12 sheets filo pastry
(preferably purchased chilled
rather than frozen)

Spray oil

Method

1. Make rissole mixture, adding the peas, sweet potato, breadcrumbs, and tomato sauce.

2. Mix very well with your hand, blending all the flavours and kneading the mixture—this helps make it more smooth and tender for cooking and gives a better end result.

3. Preheat oven to 180°C (350°F)

4. Place a sheet of pastry on benchtop, spray lightly with oil, then place a second on top, spray with oil, and finally a third sheet on top and also spray this last sheet.

5. Make a roll of some of the filling, and place on the long side of the pastry, leaving a 2-centimetre (¾-inch) gap on the edge to help with rolling. Roll up the pastry into a long roll, wet the final edge to help hold the roll together, then cut into 3-centimetre lengths and place on baking tray, folded side down. You should get 8 sausage rolls from each long roll.

6. When all the filling is used, spray all the sausage rolls with spray oil, and bake until the pastry is golden and the meat cooked through—this takes about 25–30 minutes.

7. Serve hot with tomato sauce, tomato relish, or plum sauce (see Sauces page 215).

Nutrition data per sausage roll:
277 kJ (66 cal), carbohydrate 8g, protein 5g, fat 2g, saturated fat 0.6g, fibre 1g, sodium 113mg
GI rating: med–high

Spinach triangles

**Serves 6
(2 triangles per person)
Preparation/cooking time:
40 minutes**

½ quantity Spinach and ricotta filling (see page 140)

7–8 sheets filo pastry

Spray oil

Sesame seeds (optional)

Method

1. Make filling.
2. Preheat oven to 180°C (350°F)
3. Place 1 sheet filo on bench, spray with oil, cover with a second sheet, oil this, Add a third sheet.
4. Cut into 5 equal strips along the width of the pastry.
5. Place 1½–2 tablespoons filling at one end of a pastry strip then fold over along the pastry so you shape a triangle. Place on baking sheet with last pastry fold down, then repeat with all the strips.
6. Prepare a second pastry sheet as for steps 3 and 4, fill and fold as for step 5.
7. There are 1–2 pastry sheets remaining. Depending on the amount of filling left, make further pastry strips (3 thicknesses), fill and fold as before.
8. Spray all the triangles with spray oil, sprinkle with sesame seeds and bake until golden brown and crisp. Can be reheated in oven if made ahead of time.

Nutrition data per serve:
533 kJ (128 cal), carbohydrate 10g, protein 8g, fat 6g, saturated fat 2.8g, fibre 2g, sodium 234mg
GI rating: high

Nibbles and party foods

Special occasion meals

There are many recipes in this book which can be used to create a wonderful dinner party. Here we give you a few extra special ones. We have separated them from the other recipes as we consider them mainly for special occasions as they use expensive ingredients, are a little higher in fat or are more complicated to prepare than the other recipes in this book.

Mediterranean-style mussels

Black mussels are ideal for this recipe. However, it is also excellent with clams or pipis. Green-lipped mussels are also perfect for cooking this way.

Serves 4
Preparation/cooking time:
15–20 minutes

2 teaspoons olive oil

2 medium leeks, sliced

3 large peeled tomatoes or 425g (15oz) can tomatoes, chopped

1 tablespoon no-added-salt tomato paste

¼ teaspoon ground basil

½ teaspoon ground oregano

Ground black pepper to taste

Salt to taste (optional and omit if using canned tomatoes)

1½ kg (3¼lb) mussels in shells, scrubbed and beards removed

Method

1. Heat oil in a saucepan and sauté leeks until tender.
2. Add tomatoes, tomato paste, basil, oregano, pepper and salt (if desired).
3. Bring to the boil and add mussels.
4. Cover and cook until shells open (this takes only a few minutes).
5. Serve in bowls with crusty wholegrain bread.

Nutrition data per serve:
580 kJ (139 cal), carbohydrate 9g, protein 14g, fat 4g, saturated fat 0.8g, fibre 3g, sodium 652mg
GI rating: low

Singapore noodle soup

Serves 6
Preparation/cooking time:
45 minutes

2 teaspoons sesame oil

2 cloves garlic, crushed,
or 1 teaspoon minced garlic

½ teaspoon grated
or minced fresh ginger

6 cups Basic homemade
chicken stock

300g (10½oz) green prawns,
shelled and de-veined

½ cup frozen corn

100g (3½oz) fine egg noodles

180g (6½oz) lean barbequed pork,
cut into thin strips

1 cup bean sprouts, washed
and drained

300g (10½oz) spinach leaves,
washed and dried

100g (3½oz) canned water
chestnuts, drained

1 cup Chinese broccoli

½ teaspoon 5-spice powder

8 spring onions, trimmed and
finely chopped

½ cup finely diced cucumber

Method

1. Heat oil and fry garlic and ginger until they start to brown.
2. Add the stock, prawns and corn and simmer 3 minutes.
3. Add noodles and simmer a further 5 minutes.
4. Add pork, bean sprouts, spinach, water chestnuts, broccoli and 5-spice powder and simmer 2 minutes.
5. Pour into a serving bowl and garnish with spring onions, and cucumber.

Nutrition data per serve:
864 kJ (207 cal), carbohydrate 19g, protein 22g, fat 3g,
saturated fat 0.5g, fibre 5g, sodium 217mg
GI rating: low

Gazpacho

*Although most of us associate soup with cold winter weather,
chilled soups can make a refreshing light meal or starter to a summer meal
This tangy soup can also be served hot with toasted wholegrain croutons.*

Serves 4

**Preparation/cooking time:
25 minutes**

1 small cucumber, peeled

3 spring onions

½ red capsicum

½ green capsicum

2 sticks of celery

4 medium ripe tomatoes,
or one 425g (15oz) can of tomatoes

1 medium white onion

1 cup tomato juice

1 teaspoon ground black pepper

8–10 drops tabasco sauce
(this is really hot—check soup
flavour as you add it)

Chopped parsley, for garnish

Method

1. Finely chop half the cucumber, spring onions, one ¼ of each capsicum, one stick of celery and one tomato. Set aside.
2. Roughly chop all remaining vegetables and place in food processor with tomato juice, pepper and tabasco sauce and blend until smooth.
3. Add finely chopped vegetables, mix and chill well.
4. Serve chilled, garnished with chopped parsley.

Storage: Cover and refrigerate for up to three days.

Nutrition data per serve:
283 kJ (68 cal), carbohydrate 10g, protein 4g, fat trace, saturated fat 0g, fibre 4g, sodium 234mg
GI rating: low

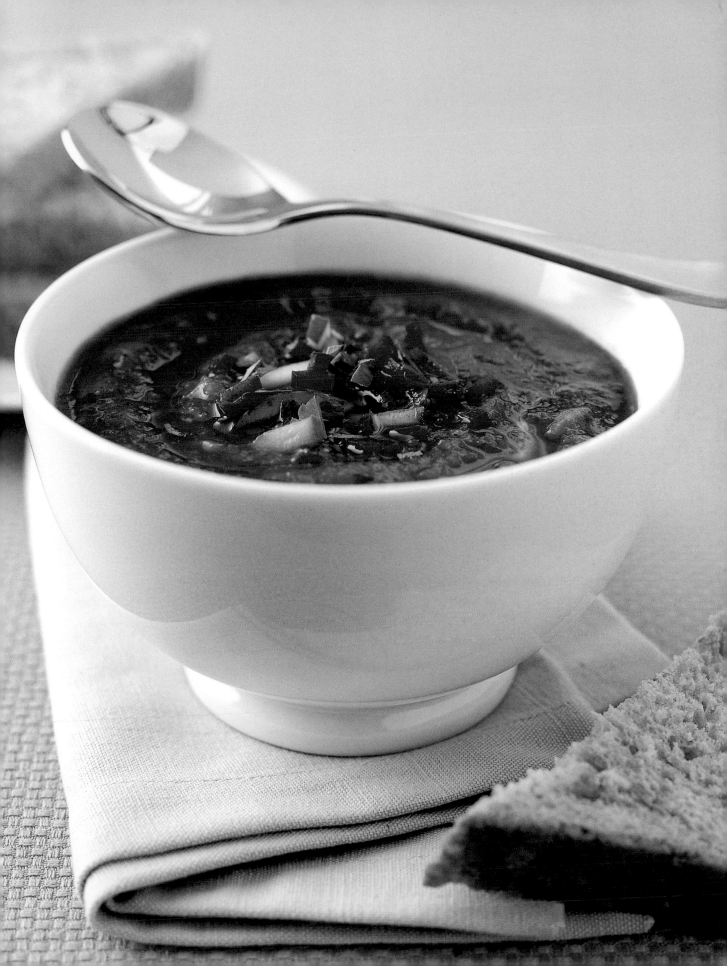

Baked beef fillet with cherry sauce

Serves 8
Preparation/cooking time:
1 hour

1kg (2¼lb) eye fillet of beef, trimmed of visible fat

2 teaspoons chopped fresh oregano or 1 teaspoon dried oregano

3 small sprigs fresh rosemary or 1 teaspoon dried rosemary

1 quantity cherry sauce

4 sprigs oregano or rosemary, for garnish

Method

1. Preheat oven to 210°C (410°F)
2. Place the beef on a large piece of aluminium foil.
3. Sprinkle with oregano and rosemary and wrap beef.
4. Place in a baking dish and bake for 30 minutes in oven.
5. Uncover and bake for a further 15 minutes.
6. Remove from oven, pour juices into bowl. Loosely cover meat with foil and let stand in a warm place.
7. Make sauce and add meat juices.
8. Cut beef into thick slices and serve topped with cherry sauce and garnished with a sprig of oregano or rosemary.

Nutrition data per serve:
1576 kJ (377 cal), carbohydrate 37g, protein 29g, fat 7g, saturated fat 2.6g, fibre 5g, sodium 129mg

Sauce
Makes 2 cups (serves 8)
Preparation/cooking time:
15 minutes

2 cups fresh ripe cherries, pitted or 300g (10½oz) frozen unsweetened cherries

½ cup chicken stock

1 teaspoon Worcestershire sauce

1 tablespoon brandy

Method

1. Place 1 cup of cherries into a saucepan or in a microwave bowl with stock and Worcestershire sauce.
2. Boil for eight minutes until cherries are soft, or microwave on high for four minutes. Puree and return to saucepan or bowl.
3. Add remaining cup of cherries and brandy. Simmer for two minutes or microwave on high for two minutes, and serve.

Nutrition data per total quantity:
906 kJ (217 cal), carbohydrate 37g, protein 3g, fat 1g, saturated fat 0g, fibre 5g, sodium 68mg
GI rating: low

Roast vegetable couscous

Serves 8
Preparation/cooking time:
60 minutes

1 medium potato, washed
and cut into 2cm (¾inch) chunks

1½ cup sweet potato, peeled
and cut into 2cm (¾inch) chunks

1 cup pumpkin, peeled
and cut into 2cm (¾inch) chunks

2 large red onions, peeled
and cut into quarters

2 tablespoons balsamic vinegar

1 tablespoon olive oil

1 teaspoon sugar

½ cup chopped dried apricots

½ cup currants

½ cup hot water

½ cup almond slivers

2 teaspoons oil

1 teaspoon curry powder

1 teaspoon ground cumin

1 teaspoon ground coriander

Pinch ground cloves

1–2 teaspoons fresh ginger, minced or grated

3 stalks celery, chopped into small cubes

1 capsicum, diced

1 tablespoon chopped fresh mint

1–2 tablespoons chopped fresh coriander
(optional)

1½ cups instant couscous

1½ cups Basic homemade chicken stock
(page 89)

Method

1. Preheat the oven to 200°C (400°F)
2. Place the chopped potato, pumpkin, sweet potato and onion in a large bowl. Add the oil, vinegar and sugar and toss together.
3. Cover a baking tray with baking paper, spread the vegetables evenly over the tray, bake until tender—about 30 minutes.
4. While the vegetables are cooking, soak the apricots and currants in the hot water.
5. Toast the almonds in the microwave until just changing colour.
6. Place the curry powder, cumin, coriander, cloves, and ginger into a large frying pan with the oil. Fry 1–2 minutes to toast the spices. Do not allow to burn.
7. Add the celery and capsicum and cook a further 3–4 minutes.
8. Add the roast vegetables, the mint and coriander, and the soaked dried fruit (with any juice), stir to combine all ingredients well, and keep warm.
9. Prepare the couscous using chicken stock in place of water. When the couscous has been fluffed up, add it to the other ingredients in the frying pan and fold all together.
10. Serve with the almonds sprinkled over.

Storage: This dish freezes well.

Nutrition data per serve:
1354kJ (324 cal), carbohydrate 50g, protein 9g, fat 8g, saturated fat 0.9g, fibre 5g, sodium 34mg
GI rating: med

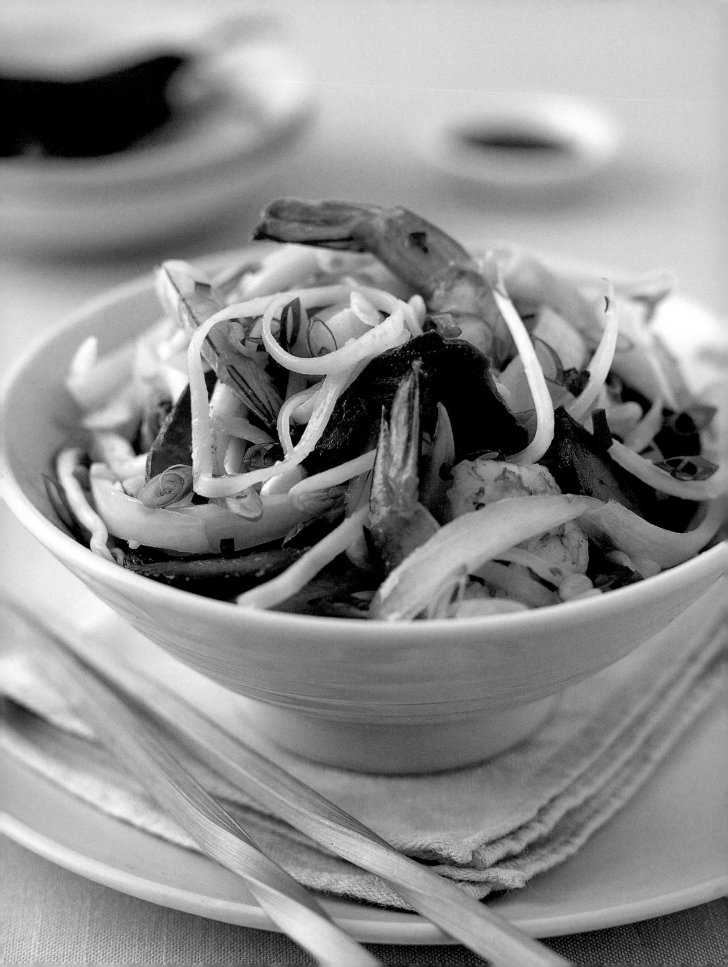

Malaysian fried rice noodles (Char kway teow)

Chinese grocery stores sell fresh rice noodles as 'sa hor fun'.
Most large supermarkets also have a range of fresh noodles.

Serves 4
Preparation/cooking time:
20 minutes

2 teaspoons oil

1 clove garlic, finely chopped

2 medium onions, cut into wedges

1–2 fresh chillies, deseeded
and chopped

100g (3½oz) lean barbecue pork,
cut into strips

150g (5¼oz) green prawns,
shelled and de-veined

150g (5¼oz) calamari (squid) rings

1 cup bean sprouts

300g (10½oz) fresh rice noodles
(char kway teow)

2 teaspoons oyster sauce

Pepper to taste

2 eggs, beaten

3 spring onions, trimmed
and chopped, for garnish

2 tablespoons chopped
coriander, for garnish

Method

1. Heat half the oil in a wok and fry garlic, onion and chilli until soft.
2. Add pork, prawns and calamari and continue cooking for two to three minutes or until seafood is cooked.
3. Add bean sprouts and toss.
4. Remove mixture from wok.
5. Add remaining oil to wok, heat and then add noodles.
6. Toss gently until heated.
7. Add oyster sauce and pepper and toss to mix.
8. Add eggs and stir until set.
9. Return pork and seafood mixture to wok, mix in well.
10. Serve hot garnished with chopped spring onions and coriander.

Nutrition data per serve:
1060 kJ (250 cal), carbohydrate 20g, protein 26g, fat 7g, saturated fat 1.6g, fibre 2g, sodium 440mg
GI rating: low

Chicken with strawberry and peppercorn sauce

Serves 4
Preparation/cooking time:
15 minutes

2 teaspoons oil

4 chicken fillets

1 quantity strawberry
and peppercorn sauce

Green beans or snow peas

Method

1. Brush the frying pan with oil and heat over medium heat. Sauté the chicken fillets until cooked and golden brown. (You can microwave them on high for three minutes but they will not brown.)

2 Prepare sauce.

3. Arrange fillets on serving plates, spoon over the sauce and serve accompanied by blanched green beans or snow peas.

Variation: Sliced turkey breast with strawberry and peppercorn sauce makes a wonderful special occasion or Christmas dinner.

Nutrition data per serve:
1064 kJ (254 cal), carbohydrate 5g, protein 30g, fat 9g, saturated fat 2.5g, fibre 1g, sodium 116mg

Sauce
Makes 2 cups
(1 serve is ½ cup)
Preparation/cooking time:
15 minutes

½ cup dry white wine

½ punnet (125g, 4½oz) strawberries, washed, hulled and pureed

2 teaspoons lemon juice

1 tablespoon brandy

2 teaspoons green or pink peppercorns

½ cup canned evaporated skim milk, chilled

Method

1. Bring wine to the boil and reduce to half by simmering.

2. Add strawberry puree, lemon juice, brandy and peppercorns.

3. Bring back to the boil, simmer for one minute and set aside to cool.

4. Whip milk until it is thick. Gradually add the strawberry mixture, whipping constantly.

5. Gently reheat the mixture, but do not allow it to boil.

6. Serve immediately.

Nutrition data per serve:
271 kJ (65 cal), carbohydrate 5g, protein 3g, fat trace, saturated fat 0g, fibre 1g, sodium 42mg
GI rating: low

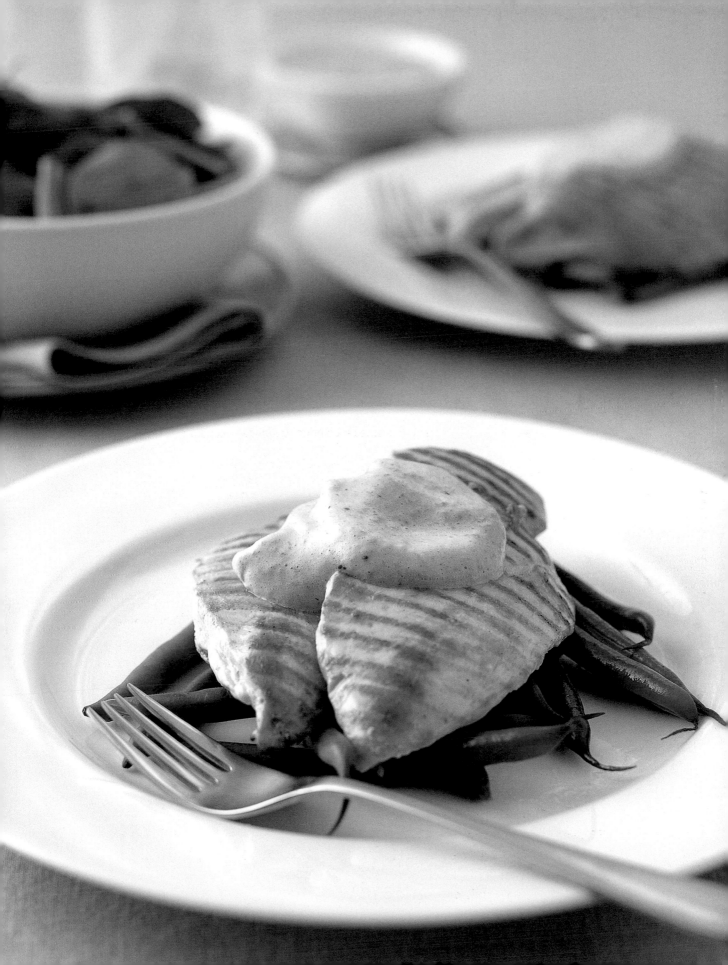

Creamy baked cheesecake

Serves 8
Preparation/cooking time:
1 hour 30 minutes

100g (3½oz) shredded wheatmeal
biscuits, crushed

2 tablespoons ground almonds
or almond meal

2 tablespoons low salt
margarine, melted

1 tablespoon water

300g (10½oz) low-fat ricotta
cheese

1 tablespoon fine semolina

125g (4½oz) low-fat
(80% fat reduced) cream cheese

⅓ cup caster sugar

3 eggs, separated

1 teaspoon grated lemon rind

2 tablespoons lemon juice

1½ cups fruit pulp (e.g. mango,
berries, apricots or other fruit)
or 1 cup passionfruit pulp

Method

1. Combine biscuit crumbs, ground almonds, melted margarine and water. Spread over the base of a lightly greased 20-centimetre (8-inch) spring-form cake tin, press down firmly, and refrigerate while mixing the filling.
2. Place ricotta cheese, semolina, cream cheese, sugar, egg yolks, lemon rind and juice, and half the fruit in a food processor or blender and process until smooth.
3. Beat egg whites until soft peaks form.
4. Fold cheese mixture into egg whites, then lightly fold the remaining fruit through the mixture. Spoon mixture into prepared tin and bake at 180°C (350°F) for 50–55 minutes or until firm. Cool in pan.

Nutrition data per serve:
1130 kJ (270 cal), carbohydrate 26g, protein 10g, fat 14g, saturated fat 4.4g, fibre 2g, sodium 168mg
GI rating: med

Flambéed crêpes

Serves 8
Preparation/cooking time:
10 minutes

1 punnet (250g, 9oz) strawberries, washed and hulled

2 bananas, sliced

8 apricots, stoned and quartered

Juice of 1 orange

½ teaspoon ground cinnamon

4 tablespoons brandy

8 Thin pancakes or crêpes (1 per serve) (see page 148), warmed

Method

1. In a frying pan, combine fruit, orange juice and cinnamon and simmer gently for approximately five minutes until fruit heats through and softens.
2. Drain off juice and set aside.
3. Add brandy to pan, heat and ignite with a match or lighter, being careful not to burn yourself. Stir gently and allow brandy to burn out.
4. Pour juice back into pan and reheat.
5. Divide fruit evenly between crêpes and roll up or fold into four to make triangles.

Nutrition data per serve:
749 kJ (179 cal), carbohydrate 25g, protein 6g, fat 3g, saturated fat 0.6g, fibre 4g, sodium 34mg
GI rating: low

Crêpes suzette

Serves 8
Preparation/cooking time:
15 minutes

4 oranges, peeled and cut into segments, pith removed

Juice of 1 orange

3 tablespoons brandy

8 Thin pancakes or crêpes (1 per serve) (see page 148), warmed

Rind of 1 orange, grated

Method

1. Poach orange segments gently in orange juice until heated through.
2. Drain off juice and set aside.
3. Add brandy to fruit in frying pan, heat and ignite with a match or a lighter. Stir fruit gently and allow brandy to burn out.
4. Pour juice back into pan and reheat.
5. Place crêpes one by one in pan, filling each with fruit, and folding each into four to make a triangle. This allows crêpes to absorb the juice.
6. Serve topped with sprinkling of orange rind.

Nutrition data per serve:
642 kJ (154 cal), carbohydrate 20g, protein 5g, fat 3g, saturated fat 0.6g, fibre 3g, sodium 32mg
GI rating: low

Fruit cake

This is perfect for special occasions such as Christmas.

**Makes twenty-four slices
(1 slice per serve)
Preparation/cooking time:
1 hour 30 minutes
+ overnight soaking**

1½ cups sultanas

1 cup raisins, chopped

½ cup canned crushed pineapple
(with juice)

2 tablespoons brandy

1 cup sieved cooked pumpkin
(no lumps)

2 eggs, beaten

¼ cup sugar

½ cup skim or low-fat milk

½ cup chopped pecans or walnuts

1 teaspoon ground cinnamon

1 teaspoon mixed spice

1 cup white self-raising flour

1 cup wholemeal self-raising flour

½ teaspoon bicarbonate of soda

Method

1. Preheat oven to 170°C (340°F)
2. Mix sultanas, raisins, pineapple and brandy. Leave to soak overnight.
3. Mix pumpkin, eggs, sugar and milk.
4. Add soaked fruit, nuts and spices, then sifted flour and bicarbonate of soda. Return bran left in sieve to flour mixture. Mix well with a wooden spoon.
5. Spoon into a lightly greased round or square 20-centimetre (8-inch) cake tin.
6. Bake in oven until cooked through and browned (approximately 1–1¼ hours). Cool on a cake rack.

Storage: Keeps in an airtight container for up to one week.

Nutrition data per slice:
575 kJ (137 cal), carbohydrate 24g, protein 3g, fat 3g, saturated fat 0.3g, fibre 2g, sodium 147mg
GI rating: med

Plum pudding

Serves 6
Preparation/cooking time:
2 hours 20 minutes
+ overnight soaking

4 tablespoons sultanas

2 tablespoons currants

3 tablespoons raisins

Rind of 1 orange, grated

½ cup grated carrot, apple
or cooked pumpkin
(or a mixture of any two)

3 tablespoons brandy

½ cup plain flour

1 teaspoon ground cinnamon

1 teaspoon mixed spice

½ teaspoon nutmeg

2 tablespoons margarine

1½ slices wholegrain bread,
crumbed

1 egg, lightly beaten

⅓ (80ml) cup skim or low-fat milk

1 teaspoon vanilla essence

1 tablespoon brown sugar
or equivalent artificial sweetener

½ teaspoon bicarbonate of soda

1 tablespoon hot water

Method

1. Soak dried fruit, orange rind and carrot (or alternative) in brandy overnight.
2. Mix flour with the spices.
3. Rub margarine into flour mixture, and add the breadcrumbs.
4. Add egg, milk, fruit mixture, vanilla, and sugar or sweetener.
5. Combine bicarbonate of soda with the hot water and mix well with all the other ingredients.
6. Pour into a greased bowl or pudding basin, cover securely, and steam for 1½–2 hours.
7. Turn out and serve with Brandy sauce (see page 226).

Nutrition data per serve:
875 kJ (209 cal), carbohydrate 29g, protein 4g, fat 6g, saturated fat 1.2g, fibre 2g, sodium 112mg
GI rating: low

Food value lists

We have included this food value chart to help you find out more about food and what's in it. Most people use a limited range of food in their day-to-day eating pattern, but we now know that eating a wide range of foods helps ensure we get a nutritious diet. This list may give you the confidence to include a wider variety of food when eating out, or at home.

We have given you the glycaemic index for individual foods where this is known and the amount of energy, carbohydrate, protein and fat in different food items. Quantities of foods have been given in 'average serves' to allow you to compare them.

The tables show the most up-to-date figures available, and are based on information supplied by the Department of Health and *The GI Factor* by Dr Jennie Brand Miller, Kaye Foster-Powell, Dr Stephen Colagiuri and Dr Anthony Leeds. Note that foods are generally rated as being low glycaemic index if their GI factor is 55 or less; intermediate or medium glycaemic index if their GI factor is between 56 and 69; and high glycaemic index if their GI factor is 70 or more.

Foods vary greatly in their nutrition content, depending on factors such as place of origin, ripeness and season. In view of this, we have rounded off all figures for nutrients to the nearest whole number and weights of foods, where appropriate, to the nearest 5g. The value of commercial products varies with brands, so remember to read labels. Use this chart as a guide only to nutrition values. Foods have been arranged according to food groups and listed alphabetically.

Abbreviations and symbols:

CHO = carbohydrate   Prot = protein   * = no value available

\# = foods with a fat level in excess of the Heart Foundation Guidelines

* = no value available

^ = data is taken from food labels and sources other than the Australian Food Composition Tables

GI figures from GI database (J Brand-Miller et al), 2008. Glucose as standard.

Australian figures used wherever available.

Gi	Foods	Serve Size	Energy Kj	Kcal	Fat gm	CHO gm	Prot gm
	Breakfast cereals						
30	All-bran™	½ cup (35g)	462	110	2	14	4
55 (ave)	Bran, oat, raw	1 tbsp (10g)	153	37	1	5	2
19	Bran, rice, extruded	1 tbsp (10g)	164	39	2	3	1
74	Bran flakes	1 cup (45g)	648	155	1	28	5
77	Coco Pops™	1 cup (45g)	703	168	1	39	2
82 (ave)	Corn flakes	1 cup (30g)	475	114	trace	25	2
42	Guardian™	¾ cup (30g)	438	105	0	20	3
58	Mini wheats (wholewheat)™	1 cup (30g)	443	106	0	21	3
56 (ave)	Muesli, untoasted, unsweetened	½ cup (50g)	733	175	8	27	5
66	Nutrigrain™	1 cup (30g)	470	112	1	21	5
59	Oats, rolled, raw (Lowan™)	1/3 cup (30g)	481	115	3	19	3
42	Oats, rolled, cooked with water	1 cup (260g)	551	132	3	22	4
65 (ave)	Oats, 1 minute / instant, cooked	1 cup (260g)	543	130	3	21	4
80	Puffed wheat	1 cup (12g)	189	45	0	8	1
83	Rice bubbles™	1 cup (30g)	464	110	0	25	2
54	Special K™	1 cup (35g)	565	134	1	24	7
64	Sultana Bran™	¾ cup (45g)	640	153	1	29	4
55	Sustain™	½ cup (45g)	710	170	1	33	4
*	Wheat flakes eg Weeties™	1 cup (30g)	436	104	1	20	3
*	Wheatgerm	2 tbsp (12g)	172	41	1	4	3
67 (ave)	Wheat flake biscuits eg Weetbix™, Vitabrits™	2 bisc. (30g)	445	107	trace	20	4
	Grains and pastas						
*	Buckwheat, raw	½ cup (50g)	773	185	1	36	6
45	Buckwheat, cooked	2/3 cup (117g)	485	116	1	23	4
*	Cracked wheat (burghul, bulgar), dry	¼ cup (45g)	266	63	0	11	2
*	Cornstarch	2 tbsp (20g)	312	75	0	18	0
65	Couscous, cooked	2/3 cup (120g)	236	56	0	11	2
*	Flour, wheat, wholemeal	½ cup (70g)	993	237	2	43	8
*	Flour, wheat, white, plain	½ cup (70g)	1038	248	1	50	8
*	Pearl barley, dry	2 tbsp (35g)	476	113	1	21	3

Gi	Foods	Serve Size	Energy Kj	Kcal	Fat gm	CHO gm	Prot gm
26 (ave)	Pearl barley, boiled	½ cup 95g	449	107	1	20	3
*	Pasta, macaroni or spaghetti, white, raw	100g	1417	339	1	68	11
40 (ave)	Pasta, macaroni, or spaghetti, white, cooked	1 cup (180g)	920	220	1	44	7
49 (ave)	Pasta, egg, boiled	1 cup (170g)	948	227	1	43	9
68	Polenta, boiled with water	1 cup (250g)	965^	231^	trace^	33^	5^
40	Rice noodles, fresh, boiled	1 cup (248g)	1034	247	1	53	5
*	Rice, brown, raw	3 tbsp (48g)	743	178	1	37	4
72	Rice, brown boiled (Sunrice™)	1 cup (180g)	1156	276	2	57	6
*	Rice, white, raw short grain	3 tbsp (50g)	727	174	0	39	3
83	Rice, white, boiled short grain	1 cup (190g)	999	239	0	53	4
54	Rice, Sunrice doongara clever rice™	1 cup (190g)	999	239	0	53	4
58	Rice, Indian basmati, doongara, boiled	1 cup (190g)	999	239	0	53	4
89	Rice, jasmine, white, steamed	1 cup (180g)	954^	228^	0^	50^	5^
69	Arborio rice, cooked	1 cup(180g)	990^	237^	6^	42^	3^
50	Mahatma™ long grain white rice, boiled	1 cup (180g)	1098^	262^	1^	56^	6^
*	Sago, dry	2 tbsp (20g)	290	69	0	17	0
*	Semolina, dry	2 tbsp (25g)	344	82	0	17	3
55	Semolina, cooked	1 cup (245g)	360	86	0	17	3
68	Taco shells (corn-based)	3 small (39g)	759	181	9	21	3
	Breads:						
70	Bread, white, regular	1 slice (32g)	327	78	1	14	3
76	Bread, wholemeal, regular	1 slice (32g)	308	74	1	12	3
43	Bread, Multigrain (50% kibbled wheat)	1 slice (34g)	348	83	1	14	3
68 (ave)	Bread, white high fibre	1 slice (28g)	264	63	1	11	2
54	Bread, Wonder White™ low GI	1slice (35)	328^	78^	1^	13^	4^
36	Bread, Burgen Soy-Lin™	1 slice (40)	405^	97^	3^	12^	6^
76	Bread, dark rye	1 slice (40g)	427	102	1	18	4

GI	Food	Serving	kJ	cal	Fat (g)	Carb (g)	Fibre (g)
54	Bread, wheat white sourdough	1 slice (25g)	260	62	1	11	2
70 (ave)	Bread roll, white	1 ave (50g)	611	146	2	27	5
75	Bread, Lebanese pita, white	1 small (46g)	537	128	1	25	4
72	Bagel, white	1 (93g)	1031	247	1	47	10
74	Bread stuffing mix	2 tbsp (20g)	303	72	1	13	3
69	Crumpet, regular	1 (50g)	397	95	0	20	3
67	Croissant	1 (67g)	1150	275	16	26	9
*	English muffin	2 halves (64g)	550	132	1	23	6
*	Matzos	1 (23g)	288	69	1	14	2
Biscuits:							
*	Crackerbread™	4 (22g)	359	86	1	16	3
*	Gingernuts	2 (22g)	380	91	3	15	1
*	Sesame wheat™	2 (14g)	260	62	3	8	1
79	Morning Coffee™	2 (16g)	303	72	3	11	1
*	Rye Cruskits™	4 (27g)	431	103	1	19	4
48	Ryvita™, sunflower seeds & oats	2 (20g)	285	68	0	12	2
*	Salada, wholemeal™	4 small (14g)	261	62	2	10	2
*	Salada, plain™	4 small (15g)	262	63	2	10	1
70	Sao™	2 (18g)	335	80	3	12	2
*	Savoy™	6 (25g)	496	117	6	15	2
62	Shredded Wheat™	2 (22g)	424	101	4	15	2
*	Thin Captains™	2 (16g)	272	65	1	11	2
*	Uneeda™	2 (22g)	400	96	3	15	2
*	Vitawheat™	4 (24g)	432	103	2	16	3
Pulses:							
40	Baked beans in tomato sauce, canned	½ cup (138g)	444	106	1	15	6
26 (ave)	Chickpeas, boiled	½ cup (80g)	334	80	0	11	5
38	Chickpeas, canned	½ cup (87g)	384	92	2	12	5
*	Haricot, borlotti beans etc, dried	1 tbsp (16g)	190	45	1	6	4
*	Lentils, dried—green/brown	1 tbsp (15g)	181	43	0	6	4
37	Lentils, cooked—green/brown	½ cup (90g)	297	71	0	9	6
42	Lentils, brown, canned, drained (Edgell's™)	½ cup (99g)	265	63	0	10	4
21	Lentils, red, split, boiled	½ cup (90g)	382^	90^	trace	16^	7^

Gi	Foods	Serve Size	Energy Kj	Kcal	Fat gm	CHO gm	Prot gm
37	4-bean mix, canned, drained (Edgell's™)	½ cup (100g)	405	97	2	14	6
31 (ave)	Red kidney beans, boiled	½ cup (90g)	328	78	0	10	7
36	Red kidney beans, canned, drained (Edgell™)	½ cup (95g)	411	98	1	14	6
*	Soya beans, raw	1 tbsp (14g)	81	19	6	0	2
14	Soya beans, canned, drained	½ cup (100g)	418	100	0	3	9
*	Split peas, raw	1 tbsp (17g)	220	53	0	8	4
25	Split peas, yellow, boiled	½ cup (90g)	245	59	0	7	6
	Fruit (edible portion)						
38 (ave)	Apple, fresh	1 (165g)	367	88	0	20	0
*	Apple, canned/stewed (no added sugar)	1 cup (200g)	396	95	0	22	0
40 (ave)	Apple juice, unsweetened	½ cup (125ml)	219	52	0	13	0
34	Apricot, fresh	3 med. (125g)	294	70	0	13	1
64	Apricot, canned in light syrup	1/2 cup (130)	230^	55^	0^	12^	1^
30	Apricot, dried	6 pieces (40g)	357	85	0	18	2
*	Avocado	¼ med. (60g)	539	129	14	0	1
47	banana	1 med. (100g)	380	91	0	20	2
*	Berries —eg:blackberry, raspberry	½ cup (100g)	206	49	0	7	1
*	blueberries	½ cup (80g)	172	41	0	9	0
*	strawberries	12 med (144g)	143	34	0	4	2
63	cherries	15 med (100g)	238	57	0	12	1
54	Custard apple, fresh	¼ whole (82g)	267	64	0	13	1
42 (ave)	Date, dried	5 whole (25g)	302	72	0	17	1
*	Fig, fresh	2 med. (100g)	189	45	0	8	1
61	Fig, dried, tenderised (Dessert Maid™)	2 whole (38g)	411	98	0	20	1
25	Grapefruit, fresh	½ (104g)	120	29	0	5	1
48	Grapefruit juice, unsweetened	½ cup (125ml)	158	38	0	8	0
46 (ave)	Grapes	1 cup (170g)	451	108	0	25	1
*	Honeydew melon	¼ med (150g)	210	50	0	10	1
58	Kiwi fruit	1 med (95g)	224	54	0	9	1

*	Lemon	1 med (58g)	67	16	0	1	0
*	Lime	1 med (30g)	27	6	0	1	0
79	Lychee, canned in syrup, drained	9 whole (90g)	271	65	0	15	1
*	Mandarin	1 med (86g)	153	36	0	7	1
51	Mango, fresh	1 small (104g)	257	61	0	13	1
43	Nectarine	2 med (130g)	224	54	0	10	1
37 (ave)	Orange	1 med (130g)	225	54	0	10	1
52 (ave)	Orange juice, unsweetened, commercial	½ cup (125ml)	181	43	0	9	1
*	Passionfruit, pulp	1 med (18g)	55	13	0	1	1
56	Pawpaw	½ sml (200g)	282	67	0	14	1
42 (ave)	Peach, fresh	1 med (100g)	143	34	0	6	1
40 (ave)	Peach, canned in natural juice	¾ cup (200g)	356	85	0	18	1
38 (ave)	Pear, fresh	1 sml (110g)	276	66	0	6	1
43	Pear, canned in natural juice	¾ cup (194g)	375	89	0	21	1
66	Pineapple, fresh	1 slice (110g)	194	46	0	9	1
49 (ave)	Pineapple, canned in natural juice	2 slice (110g)	219	52	0	11	1
46	Pineapple juice	½ cup (125ml)	229	55	0	13	0
39 (ave)	Plums	1 med (66g)	108	26	0	5	0
29	Prune, dried, pitted	4 med (32g)	269	64	0	14	1
64	Raisins	¼ cup (40g)	507	121	0	29	1
56	Sultanas	¼ cup (43g)	559	134	0	32	1
*	Rhubarb, stewed, unsweetened	½ cup (130g)	95	23	0	2	1
68	Rockmelon/cantaloupe	¼ (207g)	204	49	0	10	1
*	Tamarillo	1 med (75g)	113	27	0	3	2
76 (ave)	Watermelon	1 cup (160g)	163	39	0	8	0

Milk & dairy products

	Cheese cottage, low fat	½ cup (115g)	432	103	1	2	20
	block, low fat (7%)	30g	253	60	2	0	10
	block, low fat (18%)	30g	411	98	7	0	9
	ricotta, low fat	60g	318	76	5	1	6
	cheddar	30g	517	124	11	0	7
	cream cheese	30g	423	101	10	1	3
	cream cheese, low fat (14%)	30g	241	58	5	1	3

Gi	Foods	Serve Size	Energy Kj	Kcal	Fat gm	CHO gm	Prot gm
43	Custard, h/made—custard powder, full cream milk, sugar	½ cup (140g)	549	131	4	19	5
37	Custard Trim reduced fat™	½ cup (130g)	426	102	1	18	4
57	Ice cream regular	2 scoop (48g)	372	89	5	10	2
38 (ave)	Ice cream reduced fat (light)	2 scoop (48g)	291	70	3	9	2
32 (ave)	Milk skim	1 cup (250ml)	377	90	0	13	9
*	powder, skim	3 tbsp (33g)	485	116	0	17	12
*	evaporated skim	½ cup (135g)	424	101	0	14	11
27	reduced fat (2%)	1 cup (250ml)	564	135	3	16	11
31	full cream	1 cup (250ml)	700	167	10	12	9
*	powder, full cream	3 tbsp (27g)	551	132	7	10	7
*	evaporated, full cream	½ cup (162g)	798	191	11	14	10
40 (ave)	soy beverage, full fat	1 cup (250ml)	686	146	9	13	9
35	Yoghurt low fat, natural	1 tub (200g)	446	106	trace	12	12
*	full fat, natural	1 tub (200g)	629	150	7	10	10
32 (ave)	low fat, fruit flavoured + sugar	1 tub (200g)	640	153	trace	26	10
*	full fat, flavoured/fruit	1 tub (200g)	838	200	6	26	10
23 (ave)	non-fat, fruit + artificial sweet.	1 tub (200g)	410	98	0	12	10
	Protein foods:						
	Egg, hen	1 med (55g)	297	71	5	0	6
	Fish and seafood—fish, raw	1 fillet (100g)	427	102	2	0	20
	oysters, raw	6 (90g)	277	66	2	1	11
	prawns, boiled	100g	436	104	1	0	24
	tuna/salmon canned in brine, drained	½ cup (90g)	466	111	2	0	22
38	fish fingers, oven cooked	5 (115g)	1000	261	13	22	13
*	Meat and meat products —beef, lean, mince	120g	720	172	8	0	24
*	beef, raw, lean only	120g	630	151	5	0	25
*	ham, leg, lean	1 slice (30g)	157	38	2	0	6
*	lamb, raw, lean only	120g	712	170	7	0	26

GI	Food	Serve	kJ	Cal	Fat (g)	Carb (g)	Protein (g)
*	liver	120g	815	195	9	3	25
*	luncheon meat	1 slice (30g)	277	66	5	1	4
28	pork, raw, lean only	120g	610	146	5	0	25
*	sausages (fried)#	2 (90g)	1035	247	19	5	14
*	salami #	3 slices (42g)	748	179	16	1	9
*	veal, raw, lean only	120g	545	130	3	0	26
*	Nuts – almonds, raw	1/3 cup (60g)	1025	245	22	2	8
7	peanuts, raw	1/3 cup (46g)	1098	262	22	4	11
*	pecans, raw	1/3 cup (50g)	1238	296	30	2	4
*	walnuts, raw	1/3 cup (40g)	1216	291	29	1	6
*	pine nuts, raw	20g	584	140	14	1	3
*	peanut butter	1 tbsp (20g)	513	123	10	2	5
*	Poultry—chicken breast, no skin, raw	120g	680	163	7	0	26
*	Tofu / soy bean curd	½ cup (110g)	538	129	7	1	13
	Fats and high fat snack foods						
*	Cream, thickened #	2 tbsp (40g)	586	140	15	1	1
42	Corn chips #	50g	1081	258	15	26	4
*	Salad dressing, French #	2 tbsp (40g)	453	108	10	5	0
*	Mayonnaise, light	1 tbsp (20g)	164	39	3	4	0
*	Margarine / butter #	1 tbsp (20g)	574	137	15	0	0
*	Olives in brine	4 med. (27g)	121	29	1	0	5
*	Oil #	1 tbsp (20g)	673	161	18	0	0
57	Potato crisps #	50g	1098	263	16	24	3
72 [ave]	Popcorn (microwave cooked)	20g	475	114	9	7	1
	Sugars, confectionery, miscellaneous:						
45 [ave]	Chocolate, milk #	6 sq. (30g)	647	155	8	19	2
66	Cordial, diluted	1 cup (250ml)	390	93	0	24	0
15 [ave]	Fructose	10g	160	38	0	10	0
103 [ave]	Glucose	10g	164	38	0	10	0
50 [ave]	Honey	1 tbsp (29g)	378	90	0	24	0
78 [ave]	Jelly beans, regular	5 (15g)	203	49	0	12	1
46 [ave]	Lactose	10g	167	40	0	10	0

Gi	Foods	Serve Size	Energy Kj	Kcal	Fat gm	CHO gm	Prot gm
70	Life Savers™	10g	158	38	0	10	0
105	Maltose	10g	167	40	0	10	0
62	Mars Bar™ #	1 bar (63g)	1098	263	11	39	3
90	Real fruit bar (Uncle Toby's™)	1 bar (31g)	505	121	4	21	1
68 (ave)	Sucrose	2 tsp (10g)	167	40	0	10	0
60 (ave)	Soft drink	1 can (375ml)	657	157	0	41	0
59	Vitari™ non-dairy frozen fruit product	100ml (65g)	150	36		6	0
	Starchy vegetables (cooked, edible portion)						
63	Broad beans	½ cup (85g)	236	56	0	6	6
80 (ave)	Potato, baked, no fat added	1 sml (110g)	313	75	0	14	3
78	Potato, new, whole, boiled	5 small (175g)	460	110	0	22	4
72 (ave)	Potato, Pontiac, peeled, boiled whole (Aust)	1 small (110g)	313	75	0	15	3
74 (ave)	Potato, mashed	½ cup (123g)	349	83	0	15	3
86	Potato, instant mash (Edgell potato whip™) dry	1 cup (58g)	874	209	3	37	4
63 (ave)	French fries #	100g	1612	385	30	26	5
52	Parsnip, peeled, boiled (Aust)	½ cup (83g)	188	45	0	8	1
48	Sweet corn on the cob, boiled (Aust)	1 cob (145)	406^	96^	2^	17^	3^
56 (ave)	Sweet corn, kernels, cooked	½ cup (87g)	395	94	1	17	3
47	Sweet corn, kernels, frozen, microwaved	½ cup (87g)	395	94	1	17	3
61	Sweet potato (Aust)	½ cup (105g)	315	75	0	15	2
54	Taro, peeled, boiled	80g	351	84	0	19	2
35	Yam, peeled, boiled	½ cup (80g)	315	75	0	18	2

Low starch vegetables

Where ½ cup cooked vegetables provides **5grams of carbohydrate or less**, we have classified them as 'low starch vegetables'. These vegetables are also low in kilojoules (calories), protein and fat, but **high in vitamins, minerals, and fibre. Include them in your daily meals and snacks**—remember the guideline to include 5 serves vegetables daily.

The GI values are not determined for very low starch vegetables, as their effect on blood glucose levels is negligible. Where vegetables in this list provide some starch, the GI factor is shown in brackets.

Artichoke, globe	asparagus	bean shoots/sprouts	beans, French	beetroot (64)
Bok choy	broccoli	Brussels sprouts	cabbage	capsicum (bell
Carrot (39) ave	cauliflower	celery	Chinese broccoli	pepper)
Chinese cabbage	choko	cucumber	eggplant (aubergine)	zucchini
Endive	garlic	kale	Kohlrabi	
Lettuce	marrow	mushrooms	mung beans/sprouts	
Onion	parsley	peas (51)	pumpkin, butternut (51)	
Radish	silverbeet	spinach	summer/baby squash	
Swede (72)	tomato	turnip	watercress	

Recipe index

A

apple and sultana muffins 82
apple and sultana pancakes 76
apple scones 83
apricot and sesame pork 186
apricot chicken 180
apricot pecan muffins 82
apricot rock cakes 84
asparagus and green bean salad 206
asparagus and snow peas 200
asparagus rolls 86
avocado, spinach and orange salad 208

B

barbecue marinade 224
beans
  asparagus and green bean salad 206
  beef and bean burritos 188
  beef 'n' bean jacket potatoes 111
  broad bean and smoked salmon
    salad 116
  cheesy bean jacket potatoes 111
  mixed bean salad 119
  red curry of bean curd and beans 163
  succotash 154
beef
  beef and bean burritos 188
  beef 'n' bean jacket potatoes 111
  Bolognese sauce 138
  cannelloni 145
  curry 190
  Italian style 191
  meatballs in tomato gravy 193
  meatloaf with spicy barbecue sauce 194
  rissoles 187
  stir-fry steak with black bean sauce 129
  stroganoff 195
beetroot leaves and spinach salad 211
Bircher muesli 73
blueberry muffins 82
Bolognese sauce 138
Bombay burgers with raita 161
broad bean and smoked salmon salad 116
broccoli, lemon 202
bruschetta 98
  mushroom and herb 99
  tomato and basil 100
brussels sprouts with almonds, curried 202
burritos, beef and bean 188

C

cabbage, sweet and sour red 201
cajun fish 169
cannelloni, meat 145
cannelloni, spinach and ricotta 143
carrots, orange-glazed 201
cauliflower and sweet potato, curried 153
cheese sauce 216
cheese toast, savoury 87
cheesy bean jacket potatoes 111
chicken
  apricot chicken 180
  Chinese chicken and sweetcorn soup 95
  enchiladas 179
  pea, spinach and chicken soup 90
  satay chicken 182
  spread 86
  stir-fry 126
  stock 89
  sweet and sour stir-fry 128
  tandoori chicken 180
coleslaw 214
  jacket potatoes with 111
corn
  Chinese chicken and sweetcorn soup 95
  creamy corn pasta sauce 137
  herby corn muffins 81
  succotash 154
crêpes 148
cucumber and orange salad 208
curried brussels sprouts with almonds 202
curried pasta salad 118
curried tuna and rice casserole 172
curry
  bean curd and beans (red) 163
  beef 190
  dressing 220
  pork (green) 183
  potato, eggplant and pea (dry) 146
  sweet potato and cauliflower 153

D

dressings see also sauces
  creamy orange 221
  curry 220
  hot Thai 220
  orange and soy 221

E

eggplant neapolitan 205
eggplant, potato and pea dry curry 146
eggs 158
  French toast 77
  quick and easy quiche 108
  Spanish omelette 113
enchiladas, chicken 179

F

fettucini salmon salad 115
fish
  broad bean and smoked salmon
    salad 116
  cajun fish 169
  curried tuna and rice casserole 172
  fettucini salmon salad 115
  fish in orange sauce 170
  homemade fish and chips 177
  nicoise salad 118
  pasta marinara 173
  piquant fish in foil 168
  salmon and potato cakes 176
  salmon mornay 171
  sandwich fillings 97
  stir-fried bok choy with fish and
    almonds 175
  Thai fish cakes 178
  whole fish in ginger 170
French toast 77
fruit crunch muesli 73
fruit smoothie 74

G

gado gado 166
gnocchi, potato 147
gnocchi, semolina, with mushroom
  sauce 155
Greek lamb marinade 224
green pea soup 90

H

ham and cheese muffins 81
hamburgers in grainy rolls 101
herby corn muffins 81
homemade fish and chips 177
hot Thai dressing 220
hot Thai salad 212

I

Indian lamb in spinach sauce 196
Irish stew 197
Italian-style beef 191

J

jacket potatoes 111

K

kangaroo fillets, seared 198

L

lamb
  Greek lamb marinade 224
  Indian lamb in spinach sauce 196
  Irish stew 197
lasagne, vegetarian 142
lemon broccoli 202
lentils
  Bombay burgers with raita 161
  Middle Eastern lentil soup 94

M

mango, pork with 184
marinades 222
  barbecue 224
  Greek lamb 224
  red wine 224
  Singapore sizzler 224
meatballs in tomato gravy 193
meatloaf with spicy barbecue sauce 194
Mexican polenta pie 162
minestrone 92
mixed bean salad 119
muesli, Bircher 73
muesli, fruit crunch 73
muffin pizzas, quick 105
muffins
  apple and sultana 82
  apricot pecan 82
  basic savoury 80
  basic sweet 82
  blueberry 82
  ham and cheese 81
  herby corn 81
  raspberry 82
  sweet potato and spring onion 81
mushroom
  bruschetta, mushroom and herb 99
  pumpkin and mushrooms 200
  salad 211
  semolina gnocchi with mushroom
    sauce 155

stroganoff 110
stroganoff, jacket potatoes with 111
sun-dried tomato and mushroom
  risotto 133
vegetable skewers 205

N
nicoise salad 118
noodles 121–2
O
omelette, Spanish 113
orange and cucumber salad 208
orange and soy dressing 221
orange dressing, creamy 221
orange-glazed carrots 201
P
pancakes 148
  apple and sultana 76
  crêpes 148
  savoury fillings 150
pasta 136
  Bolognese sauce 138
  creamy corn sauce 137
  curried pasta salad 118
  fresh tomato sauce 139
  marinara 173
  meat cannelloni 145
  spinach and ricotta cannelloni 143
  spinach and ricotta sauce/filling 140
  tomato and chickpea sauce 141
  vegetarian lasagne 142
pasties 109
pastry 108
peanut (satay) sauce 216
peas
  dry curry of potato, eggplant and pea 146
  green pea soup 90
  pea, spinach and chicken soup 90
  snow peas and asparagus 200
  spiced rice with peas 135
  tomato and chickpea sauce 141
piquant fish in foil 168
pita pizza 106
pizzas 104
  pita 106
  quick muffin 105
plum 219
polenta pie, Mexican 162
pork
  apricot and sesame pork 186
  green pork curry 183
  pork with mango 184
  stir-fry 126
  sweet and sour stir-fry 128
potatoes 110, 146
  dry curry of potato, eggplant and pea 146
  gnocchi 147
  homemade fish and chips 177
  jacket potatoes 111
  roast winter vegetable medley 156
  salmon and potato cakes 176
pumpkin and mushrooms 200
pumpkin and sweet potato soup 96
Q
quiche, quick and easy 108

R
raspberry muffins 82
red wine marinade 224
relish, tomato 222
rice 121, 130
  basic risotto 130
  fried rice 134
  rice salad with roasted peanuts 114
  seafood risotto 133
  spiced rice with peas 135
  sun-dried tomato and mushroom
    risotto 133
  vegetable risotto 131
risotto
  basic 130
  meat or fish 131
  seafood 133
  sun-dried tomato and mushroom 133
  vegetable 131
rissoles 187
roast winter vegetable medley 156
S
salads 206
  asparagus and green bean 206
  avocado, spinach and orange 208
  broad bean and smoked salmon 116
  curried pasta 118
  fettucini salmon 115
  high carb 114
  hot Thai 212
  mixed bean 119
  mushroom 211
  nicoise 118
  orange and cucumber 208
  rice salad with roasted peanuts 114
  spinach and beetroot leaves 211
  spinach Valentino 212
  sweet potato 151
  tabbouleh 209
  tossed 206
salmon and potato cakes 176
salmon fettucini salad 115
salmon mornay 171
sandwich fillings 97–8
satay chicken 182
satay (peanut) sauce 216
sauces see also dressings
  cheese 216
  plum 219
  satay (peanut) 216
  sweet and sour 217
  white 215
scones, apple 83
seafood stir-fry 125
seafood risotto 133
semolina gnocchi with mushroom
  sauce 155
Singapore sizzler marinade 224
snow peas and asparagus 200
soups 88–96
  basic chicken stock 89
  Chinese chicken and sweetcorn 95
  green pea 90
  Middle Eastern lentil 94
  minestrone 92
  old fashioned veggie 91

pea, spinach and chicken 90
pumpkin and sweet potato 96
Spanish omelette 113
spiced rice with peas 135
spinach
  avocado, spinach and orange salad 208
  Indian lamb in spinach sauce 196
  pea, spinach and chicken soup 90
  pie 165
  spinach and beetroot leaves salad 211
  spinach and ricotta cannelloni 143
  spinach and ricotta pasta sauce/
    filling 140
  Valentino 212
stir-frys 120–1
  bok choy with fish and almonds 175
  chicken 126
  flavours for 123
  pork 126
  seafood 125
  steak with black bean sauce 129
  sweet and sour pork or chicken 128
stroganoff, beef 195
stroganoff, mushroom 110
  jacket potatoes with 111
succotash 154
sukiyaki, tofu 164
sun-dried tomato and mushroom risotto 133
sweet and sour pork or chicken 128
sweet and sour red cabbage 201
sweet and sour sauce 217
sweet potato
  curried sweet potato and cauliflower 153
  salad 151
  pumpkin and sweet potato soup 96
  roast winter vegetable medley 156
  sweet potato and spring onion muffins 81
T
tabbouleh 209
tandoori chicken 180
Thai dressing, hot 220
Thai fish cakes 178
Thai salad, hot 212
toast, savoury cheese 87
tofu (bean curd) and beans red curry 163
tofu sukiyaki 164
tomato
  fresh tomato pasta sauce 139
  meatballs in tomato gravy 193
  relish 222
  sun-dried tomato and mushroom
    risotto 133
  tomato and basil bruschetta 100
  tomato and chickpea pasta sauce 141
  vegetable skewers 205
  zucchini and tomato lavash bake 103
tuna and rice casserole, curried 172
V
vegetable nut loaf 159
vegetable skewers 205
vegetarian lasagne 142
veggie soup, old fashioned 91
W
white sauce 215
Z
zucchini and tomato lavash bake 103
zucchini creole 200

Index

A

Accredited Practising Dietitians (APD) 9
adolescents 46–8
alcohol 32–3
  diet beers 32
  hypoglycaemia and 39
  low alcohol beers 32
  older people 50
  reacting with medication 33
  standard drinks 33
  teenagers 47
alternative names for foods 70–1
artificial sweeteners 45, 67, 69
Australian Dietary Guidelines see Dietary
  guidelines

B

blood glucose level
  exercise and 53
  glycaemic index and 23
  glycosylated haemoglobin (HbA1c)
    blood test 17
  high (hyperglycaemia) 8–9, 15
  low (hypoglycaemia) 39–42
  monitoring 16–17
  sugars and starches increasing 21
  weight management and 16
bread and cereals 21, 78
  eating out 58
  gluten free diet 44
  sandwich fillings 97
  snacks 78
breakfast 72
  recipes 73–7

C

calcium 32, 50
  older people 50
  soy milk 52
  vegetarian diet 52
carbohydrates 19–20, 21
  added sugars 24–5
  balanced eating 130
  breakfast 72
  coeliac disease and 43
  fibre 19, 24
  foods rich in 8
  glucose made from 7
  gluten free 43–4
  glycaemic index (GI) 22–4
  hypoglycaemia and 39–42
  illness, during 38
  pregnancy 45
  starches 7–8, 19, 21
  sugar see Sugar
cereals 21, 72, 78
cheese 31, 69, 97, 158
  sandwich fillings 97
children 46–8
  encouraging healthy eating 46
  lunch ideas 48
  managing diabetes away from home 48
  participating in diabetes management 47
  snacking 47
Chinese food 58

cholesterol 27–9
  food labels 66
  good and bad 28
coconut milk 69
coeliac disease 42–5
  carbohydrates suitable for 43–4
  hypoglycaemia 45
  management 44–5
Credentialled Diabetes Educators (CDEs) 9

D

dairy products 31, 32, 50
dehydration 39
Diabetes Australia 9
diabetes insipidus 10
diabetes mellitus 7
  diagnosing 14
  increasing incidence 7
  information about 9
  management of 15–54
  medication 36–7
  types 10–13
  what is 7
diagnosing diabetes 11, 14
  early diagnosis 15
diarrhoea 39
Dietary Guidelines 18–36
  alcohol 32–3
  bread and cereals 21
  carbohydrates 19–21
  dairy products 31, 32
  eggs 31, 158
  fats 26–31
  fibre 19, 24
  fish 30, 168
  fruit 21
  legumes (pulses) 20, 31, 158
  meat and poultry 30, 179
  nuts and seeds 31, 158
  protein 30, 158
  tofu 31, 158
  vegetables 20, 199
  vegetarians 50–3
  water 25

E

eating to suit your needs 56–61
eating out 56–9
eggs 31, 158
  sandwich fillings 98
exercise 16, 53–5
  blood glucose level and 53–4
  hyperglycaemia and 54
  hypoglycaemia and 54
eyes
  loss of vision 15
  regular checks 17

F

fats 26–31, 68
  cholesterol 27–9
  food labels 62
  healthy use of 28
  heart disease and 28
  high blood fat level 30
  major sources 26

margarine 69
  monounsaturated 27, 29
  omega 3 fats 28, 29
  omega 6 fats 29
  polyunsaturated 27, 29
  recipes, use in 68–9
  recommended intake 26
  reducing intake of 34
  saturated 26, 29
  stir-frys 124
  trans fats 30
  triglycerides 29
feet
  loss of feeling 15
  regular checks 17
fibre 19, 24
  breakfast 72
  food labels 62
  gluten free diet 44
  preventing constipation 49
fish 30, 168
  omega 3 fats 28, 29
  recipes 168–78
  sandwich fillings 97
flavours 123, 215
food
  alternative names 70–1
  children and adolescents 46
  Dietary Guidelines see Dietary Guidelines
  eating out 56–9
  eating to suit your needs 56–61
  labels see Food labels
  measuring 69–70
  nutrients in 18
  occasional treats 59–60
  shift work and 61
  takeaways 59
  travelling 60
  vegetarians 50–3
food labels 62–7
  all natural 67
  carbohydrate modified 67
  cholesterol-free/low cholesterol 66
  diabetic 67
  GI symbol 64
  Heart Foundation Tick 66
  healthy choices 63, 64
  ingredients list 62
  light/lite 66
  low joule 66
  nutrition panel 63
  packaging claims 64–7
  percentage fat-free 66
  sugar-free/no added sugar 6
fruit 21, 72, 78

G

gestational diabetes 10, 12–13, 45
  diagnosis 14
  risk factors 13
  type 2 diabetes developing after 13, 45
glucose 7
  body's use of 8
  insulin and 8

level in blood *see* Blood glucose level
gluten free carbohydrates 43–4
glycaemic index (GI) 22–4
  blood glucose level and 23
  classification of carbohydrates 23
  factors affecting 22
  fibre 24
  food labels 64
  GI value of recipes 68
  low GI foods 23, 78
  pasta 136
  rice 23, 121
glycosylated haemoglobin (HbA1c)
    blood test 17
Greek food 58

H
heart disease
  diabetes complication 15
  fats and 28, 29
  low-fat diet for older people 48
  poor sleep 30
  risk factors 29–30
  smoking and 30
high blood pressure and salt 34
high density lipoprotein cholesterol
    (HDL-C) 28
hyperglycaemia 9, 11
  coeliac disease and 43
  damage to body 15
  exercise and 54
  symptoms 8–9
hypoglycaemia 39–42
  carrying card with information on 41
  causes 39
  children 46, 48
  coeliac disease and 43
  eating carbohydrates for 40
  exercise and 54
  medical treatment 41
  symptoms 40
  unconsciousness 41

I
illness and diabetes 37–9
impaired fasting glucose (IFG) 10, 13
  diagnosis 14
  risk factors 13
impaired glucose tolerance (IGT) 10, 13
  diagnosis 14
  risk factors 13
Indian food 58
insulin 7, 8
  diabetes management 36–7
  discovery of 7
  dose adjustment for normal eating
    (DAFNE) 37
  insufficient production of 10, 11
  pregnancy, during 45
  purpose of 8
  rapid-onset 37
  too much *see* Hypoglycaemia
  types 36
insulin insufficiency 11
insulin resistance 11
iron in vegetarian diet 52
Italian food 59

J
Japanese food 59
K
ketosis 45
kidney disease 15
kilojoule intake 34
L
legumes 20, 31, 158
long term complications of diabetes 15
low density lipoprotein cholesterol
    (LDL-C) 28
M
management of diabetes 15–54
  asking questions 18
  children and adolescents 46–8
  diet 18–36
  exercise 16
  medication 36–7
  monitoring blood glucose 16–17
  older people 48–50
  regular health checks 17–18
  weight management 16, 33–6
margarine 69
measuring foods 69–70
meat and poultry 30, 179
  recipes 179–98
  sandwich fillings 98
medication
  alcohol reacting with 33
  illness, taking during 38
  insulin 36–7
  tablets 36
  taste of food, affecting 49
Mexican food 59
milk and milk products 31, 32, 78
  fat content 69
  snacks 78
  soy milk 52
  vegetarian diet 52
minerals 20
  carbohydrates providing 19
  vegetables providing 20, 199
  vegetarian diet 50, 52
monitoring blood glucose 16–17
N
National Diabetes Services Scheme
    (NDSS) 9
noodles 121–2
nutrients in foods 18
  nutrient value of recipes 68
  vegetarian diet 50
nuts and seeds 31, 158
O
older people 48–50
  calcium 50
  high fibre foods 49
  home meal delivery 50
  loss of appetite 49
  low-fat diet 48
  salt intake 50
  vitamin D 50
omega 3 fats 28, 29
omega 6 fats 29
Oral Glucose Tolerance Test (OGTT) 14
oven temperatures 70
overweight 11, 13

P
pancreas 8, 10, 11
pasta 136
  low GI 136
  recipes 137–45
phytochemicals 21
pregnancy 45–6
  artificial sweeteners 45
  carbohydrate intake 45
  gestational diabetes 10, 12–13, 14, 45
  ketosis risk 45
protein 30, 158
  stir-frys 122
  vegetarian diet 52, 158–66
pulses 20, 31, 158
R
restaurants, eating in 56–9
rice 121
  low GI 23, 121
  recipes 130–5
S
salt 34–5, 68
  food labels 62
  recipes, use in 68
  reducing intake 35, 50
  stir-frys 124
sandwich fillings 97
shift work and eating 61
sleep, poor, and heart disease 30
smoking and heart disease 30
snacks 78
  children 47
  recipes 79–87
soups 88
  recipes 89–96
soy milk 52
sport 53–5
starches 7–8, 19, 21
  see also Carbohydrates
  blood glucose level increased by 21
  foods rich in 8
  glucose made from 7
stir-frys 120–1
sugar 7–8, 19, 21, 69
  see also Carbohydrates
  added sugars 24–5
  artificial sweeteners 45, 67, 69
  blood glucose level increased by 21
  cutting down on 25
  food labels 62, 66
  foods rich in 8
  glucose made from 7
  recipes, use in 69
T
takeaway food 59
teenagers 47–8
teeth 17
Thai food 59
tofu 31, 158
travel and eating 60
Type 1 diabetes 10–11
  coeliac disease and 42
  diagnosis 14
  exercise and insulin 54
  risk factors 11
  treatment 11

Type 2 diabetes 10, 11–12
    coeliac disease and 42
    diagnosis 11, 14
    gestational diabetes, developing
        after 13, 45
    insulin insufficiency 11
    insulin resistance 11
    risk factors 11
    treatment 12
V
vegetables 20, 199
    recipes 200–14
    sandwich fillings 98
    stir-frys 122
vegetarians 50–3
    lacto-ovo diet 50, 52
    meatless dishes 158–66
    sources of nutrients 52
    soy milk 52
    vegan diet 50, 52
vision, loss of 15
vitamins 20
    carbohydrates providing 19
    fat-soluble 20
    older people 50
    vegetables providing 20, 199
    vegetarian diet 50, 52
    water-soluble 20
vomiting 39
W
water 25
weight management 16, 33–6
Y
yoghurt 31, 69